Even the Dar[k]

The Depths of a Father's Love

While every precaution has been taken in the preparation of this book, the publisher assumes no responsibility for errors or omissions, or for damages resulting from the use of the information contained herein.

EVEN THE DARKEST NIGHT WILL END

First edition. February 25, 2023.

Copyright © 2023 Seymond Perry, Sr..

ISBN: 979-8215302361

Written by Seymond Perry, Sr..

"Even the darkest night will end and the sun will rise."
— Victor Hugo, Les Misérables

FOR HIS ANGER IS BUT for a moment, His favor is for a lifetime. Weeping may endure for a night, but a shout of joy comes in the morning (Proverbs 30:5 AMP).

Table of Contents

Dedication 4

Acknowledgments 6

Introduction 8

Chapter 1 | Into the Valley 11

Chapter 2 | Stand as a Soldier 19

Chapter 3 | I Always Win 28

Chapter 4 | The Lernaean Hydra 36

Chapter 5 | Lay Down Your Life 47

Chapter 6 | We're Going to Make It 56

Chapter 7 | Hope Against Hope 66

Chapter 8 | The Darkest Night 78

Chapter 9 | To the Bitter End 88

Closing 99

SEYMOND PERRY, SR.

Appendix 104

Works Cited 117

Dedication

I wholeheartedly sanctify this work to the use of my Lord and Savior, Jesus Christ. He alone has given us strength to endure an onslaught of demonic aggression and attacks from the adversary, Satan. Jesus has made human repentance and spiritual resurrection possible. Because of the Redeemer's incredible offering on Calvary, we have the knowledge and the authority to stand against all opposition. Because of the blood of the Lamb, we have been healed and made whole from all hurt, lack, pain, sickness, and disease. Because of His tremendous sacrifice, we overcome, win, and always come out victorious. He has become the center of my life, and with Him as my nearest and dearest friend, I have the courage and tenacity to cast out all fear and continually march forward in faith.

Her support of my many crazy ideas over the years (stock broker, gym owner, insurance agent, personal trainer, author, etc.) is astonishing. She has been a fantastic mother to our kids. Most importantly, Sarah loves the Lord and has brought me closer to Him. And so, this book is also devoted to my wife, who fought alongside me for our son, for our family's wholeness, and our never-ending testimony on the earth. Her silent strength allowed me to stand boldly against countless doctor's reports, physical symptoms, and voices of doubt and fear in my mind. Her comfort eased the burden and responsibility that comes with manhood, fatherhood, and parenting. Because my wife refused to quit, I too found the wherewithal to press on for the prize of the high calling that is found in our Savior.

This book is devoted to the loving memory of my beautiful son, my first son, Seymond Dontre' Perry, Jr. I have oftentimes sought perfection as a parent but you have taught me that I only needed to

SEYMOND PERRY, SR.

be me. Donte, you have trained me in so many ways; you are the one who taught me how to let my guard down and love again. You are the one who taught me how to give, how to sacrifice, and how to provide expecting nothing in return. I thoroughly appreciate who you are and what you have meant to my life. Thank you for teaching me that there is more to discipline than spanking. Because of your life and testimony, I now understand how God the Father feels about me, and how he feels about all of His children.

Intense shock, confusion, disbelief, and even denial flood a person after the passing of a child. It can become almost impossible to face daily tasks or even get out of bed when you're being crushed and overwhelmed with sadness and despair. For that reason, for any person who knows the pain of losing a child, we set this book aside just for you. Take courage; the Lord, the Righteous Judge, the Holy One of Israel, sees your tears and knows your pain. He also knows the pain of watching His Son suffer and die a gruesome death. Jesus knows what you are feeling and going through, for He was a man of sorrow and well acquainted with grief. Run to Him; press into His presence and lay before Him with a broken and remorseful heart. For in the presence of the True Vine is the fullness of joy; at His right hand, there are pleasures forever. When you continually abode with the Lord, there is unmatched strength available to you; there is undying hope in the presence of the Lord. Hope for the pains of yesterday, hope for the struggles of today, hope that even the darkest night will end and the sun will rise again.

Acknowledgments

After years of church hurt, disappointing pastors, and leadership abandonment, the Head of the Church faithfully led me to a person who would protect me with the heart of the Good Shepherd. Rev. Charles W. Quann says "The most important characteristic of any pastor is a heart for God, a deep desire to live for Christ and to see others come to know him and serve him". I thank the Lord daily for Pastor Alvin Robertson (Kingdom of God Ministries-Pine Bluff). Through his dedication to accurately teaching the Word of God, my family has gained the knowledge and ability to weather the numerous storms of life boldly. Not only have Pastor Robertson's teachings been transformational to our lifestyle, but his conduct and character in private and public have also been a true model for success. We pronounce the favor and blessings of the Highest God upon him and his entire family. We speak life and wholeness over everything concerning his life; we declare his latter days will be greater than his former, in Jesus' name.

Established in 1912, Arkansas Children's Hospital offers a service to the state of Arkansas that is unmatched. Crossing various landmarks, medical establishments play a huge role in the social and economic health of practically all cities, in some instances even states. Truly the heart of God is forever towards children (Matthew 19:14); because of this, the heart of God must certainly be towards Arkansas Children's Hospital. They were designed to give optimal care to infants, children, adolescents, and their specific medical needs. In their many years of existence, countless lives have been touched, affected, and forever changed for the better. Because of their tireless efforts to bring healing

SEYMOND PERRY, SR.

and restoration to the children of this great state. We thank you for your unwavering labor of love.

Being a great physician takes more than high test scores and in-depth knowledge of medical jargon. Good doctors are consistently good communicators, organized, empathetic, curious, and possess excellent bedside manners. Dr. Beth Littrell embodies all of these qualities and so many more. She was Dontre's primary doctor from beginning to end. One characteristic that I found most impressive was her ability to advocate for Dontre's voice as well as the voice of his parents. In all sincerity, who could have asked for a better, more qualified doctor? Always kind, caring, and concerned, she was truly sent by God to serve and watch over our family. We acknowledge that humanity is flawed, weak, frail, and limited. We also recognize that this excellent doctor went above and beyond the call of duty for our household. The Perry family personally extends a heartfelt thank you to Dr. Beth for her affectionate courtesy and kindness toward our family. Because your work is beyond difficult, we will continually lift you in prayer. You will never be forgotten and will always hold a special place to win our hearts and minds.

Time would fail me, and pages would cease to exist to explain the treasure I have found in my deacon, my brother, and my closest friend, Deacon Aaron Spencer. He has always been a listening ear, a source of laughter in the depths of despair, and an encouragement when all hope was lost. Over the many years of our friendship, Aaron has become my go-to person for Biblical discussion. He has become my accountability partner and the one who encourages me to grow to higher heights and deeper depths in the Lord. I thank Christ for the invaluable companion He has graciously placed in my life. It is through the prayers, lifestyle, and faithfulness of Aaron that I was led to receive the baptism in the Holy Ghost. Come hell or high water, I've got your back. Whether a natural threat or a spiritual battle, I will always be in your corner

EVEN THE DARKEST NIGHT WILL END

rooting for you and fighting alongside you. Come what may, I will always be proud to call you my brother.

Introduction

No one is exempt from the storms of life. You will find yourself in one of three circumstances: heading into a storm, going through a storm, or coming out of a storm. But just as the disciples discovered, the storms we face can bring us to a deeper knowledge and appreciation for God. Through our various trials, we can learn that no storm is big enough to prevent God from accomplishing His perfect will in our lives. But where exactly do these problems and issues come from? How can we minimize or even do away with them altogether? One author writes: "What leads to fighting and conflicts among you? Don't they come from your desires that wage war within you? You are jealous and crave what others have and your goals go unfulfilled; so you take your frustrations out on those around you. You are envious and cannot obtain the object of your envy; so, you fight and battle."

Man, who is born of a woman, is short-lived and full of turmoil (Job 14:1 AMP).

This is life in a nutshell. No matter how perfect you believe your life to be, you will face problem after problem. These problems persistently exist and they will not move by themselves; they will only be moved when you face them and solve them. The writer of Ecclesiastes writes that life is vain, meaningless, and pointless. Because of this, he sums up the entire book with this statement: *Worship God and keep God's commandments because this is what everyone must do* (Ecclesiastes 12:13 CEB). Sachin Ramdas Bharatiya writes: "Problems in life occur only because we act without thinking or we just keep thinking without taking any action. Do not tell everyone about your problems, because not everyone has medicine in their house, but salt is there. Only when there are problems in life will you enjoy success."

SEYMOND PERRY, SR.

As far as I can tell, problems, troubles, storms, and challenges are a huge part of what makes life meaningful.

"Life will always be filled with challenges. Obstacles are part of your life so don't wait for the 'dust to settle'. Embrace the 'problems' because they are your growth, your life." - Patty Kogutek

It's the rain that helps us enjoy the sunshine; it's the winter's cold that helps us thrive in the warmth of summer; it's the depths of sadness and despair in the valley that helps us cherish the mountaintop accomplishments. While traveling through life, we will come across plenty of obstacles and issues that will attempt to distract us from the "straight and narrow" path. Oftentimes, we feel as if we don't have everything we need to deal with these issues. But if you can gain a different and better perspective of what you're facing, you can certainly make progress. And once you have a clear view of what the true problem is in your life, you can handle it much better.

Because of all of the aforementioned truths, there had to be some level of struggle within a fifteen-year-old marriage. We married young, shared good and bad times, created a family, had fights, and disagreements, and even experienced the proverbial sex drought. Surely there was trouble experienced within a fifteen-year-old marriage, most self-inflicted, but trouble nonetheless. From lies to drugs, from sexual perversion to infidelity, from lack of resources to the misuse of resources, our marriage had certainly seen it. There were times we felt so alone even within each other's company, each party experienced seasons of depression and deep isolation. Sarah and I had encountered it all, at least that's what we thought. And after clawing and fighting to regain some level of godliness and regularity in our marriage, we were finally in a "good" place. This is not to say that we had finally arrived or that we were perfect, but things were finally clearly better; life was tolerable. Despite it all, there was some hope for marriage, our children, and our careers. Our faith was steadily increasing and becoming far better than we could have ever imagined. There was finally hope for

EVEN THE DARKEST NIGHT WILL END

a better marriage, a better us; there was finally hope for a better tomorrow.

Chapter 1
Into the Valley

Then Caleb quieted the people before Moses, and said, "Let us go up at once and take possession of it; for we will certainly conquer it." *31 But the men who had gone up with him said, "We are not able to go up against the people [of Canaan], for they are too strong for us." 32 So they gave the Israelites a bad report about the land which they had spied out, saying....* (Numbers 13:30 - 32 AMP).

Numerous individuals respond differently to demanding and stressful situations. With the rapid spread of Covid-19 around the world, many people are experiencing feelings of doubt, worry, panic, and even anger. Along with these emotions, having to remain sheltered in place can produce even greater feelings of anxiousness, loneliness, boredom, and even high levels of frustration. Despite the thoughts, feelings, and concerns of the world at large, the quarantine gave my family a much-needed break from the mundane hustle and bustle of life. To work from home, to spend quality moments with my wife and children, and to seek the Lord's presence are invaluable and cherished commodities. I'm not always able to fully engage in all of these important areas of my life, at least not to the extent that I would like to. But for once, with the world at a standstill, I can fully immerse myself in the Holy Spirit and within my household. My family was safe and sound in our home, with no signs of sickness or infection. As far as we could tell, everything and everyone was well and happy. What else could a man ask for? After many years of conflict, battle, and chaos, there was finally a time of satisfaction where peace flowed through our

SEYMOND PERRY, SR.

home like a river. Although our past was scared by the many delicate and strenuous seasons, our marriage was finally beginning to flourish and blossom. But what is harmony and tranquility if it is not guarded, protected, and fought for? What is peace if one is not willing to pay the highest price? What is serenity and composure without some looming threat of danger and conflict? I used to wonder what the Redeemer meant by resisting to the point of blood. What He is saying is: Have you fought to the point where it will cost you your lives? Honestly, most of us don't desire those moments and will never be placed in those kinds of situations. But everything around us, our homes, our families, our mental health, and even our salvation have been provided to us at a cost. And the price for continued peace is love, love is what causes us to shed our blood to lay down our lives so others may live.

All good fathers desire to pass on skills, talents, and abilities to their children. Part of it may be pride and arrogance but for the most part, this deep-seated passion comes from a place of love. The Lord has graced me to be talented in many areas, from typing to reading, from teaching to leadership. Playing high school football, I developed a deep devotion to health and physical fitness. Because of this, over the years one of my favorite pastimes has become exercising; I most notably love weight lifting. Passing on to my children some of the skills that I've acquired has been a dream since each of them was born. During this season of solace Dontre' (my oldest son) and I began to exercise together. We kicked off this momentous event at one of our local gyms, slowly but steadily making progress. I will never forget the look of joy and pride on his face knowing he was making his father proud, knowing he was following in his dad's footsteps; those moments were priceless. But as Covid spread throughout the nation and the world, our local gym would eventually close. Because there's nothing more powerful than a made-up mind, I was determined to keep us moving forward. I dusted off all of my old workout equipment in the garage, pulled it outside and we continued our father/son training at home.

EVEN THE DARKEST NIGHT WILL END

IT'S SAD TO SAY BUT adults are very poor judges of when children are not being truthful. It's even sadder that parents do even worse at telling if their children are lying. Probably because, as parents, we are exposed to all of the negative situations our children engage in. From fighting to stealing, we get it all. And my loving Dontre' was no different, he was a typical child with a typical childhood. So, as time progressed in our workout sessions, he began complaining of lingering soreness and pain. As a father, I assumed that it was from the workouts or that he was being lazy, or that he was outright lying, but the discomfort and unpleasantness persisted. He and I took a few days off from working out, believing this course of action would rectify the issue. Nonetheless, after this period of rest, he was still complaining of numbness and lasting pain. Once again, presuming that maybe he pulled a muscle, I recommended he use ice packs, rest, and pain relief medications. Now his mother, on the other hand, had a certain kind of intuition about the situation. It's probably something God builds into mothers but she felt that there was a deeper issue. But like any loving wife, she trusts my judgment, especially in the area of health and fitness. After my knowledge and expertise were exhausted, the issues remained. To no avail, the pain continued, even interrupting his rest and normal function in life. The recliner was the only way he could find relief at night; this was the only way he could find anything close to good sleep. As the weeks progressed, Dontre' would complain of increasing numbness in his arm, something I was well aware of from old football injuries. I speculated a pinched nerve or poor circulation was the main culprit. Eventually, Sarah would take him to Arkansas Children's Hospital for an extensive examination. Almost immediately, the hospital staff began running a series of tests and initially could not find any issues. Even still, I'm completely positive and fully believe in the best results or at least nothing life-threatening. I even remember

SEYMOND PERRY, SR.

telling Sarah: "No news is good news." If they can't find anything then everything must be alright.

One of the most taxing parts of having any medical test is waiting for the results. It's almost impossible not to imagine the worst outcome, especially when the reports are about someone you love. When all the tests had been run and when all the screenings had been surveyed, with great trepidation, Sarah relayed to me the "bad report" that the doctors found a sizable tumor lodged between Dontre's chest and shoulder. As challenging as it can be to receive disappointing news like this, I force myself to remain positive and to think optimistically. I still believe in the best outcome and that the tumor is benign (tumors that stay in their primary location without spreading to other parts of the body), but that was not the truth we would soon have to accept. "The word "truth" in Greek means "the reality lying at the basis of an appearance; the manifested, the actual essence of a matter". It means absolute reality; it is "true" and "real." (From Faith to Faith - Watchman Nee). Although it may be difficult and almost impossible to acknowledge, the truth is that my son has now been diagnosed with cancer and the tumor is malignant. The doctors inform us that the location of the tumor makes it very difficult and almost unthinkable to perform surgery. The best course of action for Dontre's overall health and recovery is to administer chemotherapy and radiation. Chemo and radiation can be almost unbearable to full-grown adults; this is a child that will have to endure the onslaught of side effects, ailments, and symptoms. And as difficult as this may be on his young body, this course of action will give us the best possible outcome moving forward. If all of this heartbreaking information was not enough, tests reveal that Dontre' has an adult form of cancer. Almost unpronounceable to even the smartest of people: Adenocarcinoma is the name. In the coming months, we would become very familiar with and almost accepting of this fear-inducing name. Unknown to us at the time, adenocarcinoma of the lungs is rather forceful and aggressive. We did not know the

EVEN THE DARKEST NIGHT WILL END

statistics at the moment but even early diagnosis offers only a 61% chance of survival five years later. This rare cancer in adults is practically unheard of in children. To give you a point of reference, primary lung cancer in children is extremely rare, estimated to be 1 in 2 million of all childhood tumors.

It's almost inevitable that at some point in your life you'll have to deal with a scary diagnosis from a doctor. Whether it's being diagnosed with cancer, diabetes, or heart disease, most of us have gone through these life-altering situations. I guess I'm the unusual one because I've never had so much as a broken bone. But now my child, at the age of 13, has been found with a tumor. Once reality finally sets in, you wonder how your life will change. I'm concerned about what his treatments will be like. As the provider, I wonder how we will pay for all these medical expenses. And thoughts of him dying to try to creep into my mind as well. It's easy to read a list of "Five Things to Do in a Crisis", but when you're face-to-face with this news and you're afraid, all the self-help literature quickly vacates your brain. Because of the dark and dismal valley that lay before us, there was no doubt in our minds that if Jehovah Rapha did not heal Dontre', he would not be healed. To put it mildly, it can be tough for a grownup to deal with the threat of cancer; needless to say, it can be a devastating blow to parents when a child is involved. Shortly after his diagnosis, the family is still waiting on information about his condition and his treatment plan. It's hard not to have thoughts about the future and all of the "What if" scenarios. Individuals are referred to as "cancer survivors" because similar to war-scared soldiers, cancer creates an immediate crisis that produces instant wounds and scars.

Leo Tolstoy says that "even in the valley of the shadow of death, two and two do not make six." And that is almost impossible for a person like me to accept (a robotic, well-calculated, methodical, systematic person like me). If one and one don't make two, how can I win? And if they don't equal two, what do they equal? Would someone

SEYMOND PERRY, SR.

please let me know so I can be successful in this situation? Isn't that the point, to win? At all costs, whatever it takes, am I not supposed to overcome and succeed at everything I do? What is a person supposed to do when life doesn't make sense? Financial hardships. A loved one dies. Friendships wane. A job is lost. Whether it's the seasoned saint facing retirement or the high school graduate facing the burdens and pressures of an uncertain future, crisis and suffering have a way of rattling even the most confident Christian. My son has been diagnosed with cancer. Although it doesn't make any sense, I am still determined to win. I haven't developed a plan just yet and I don't know what I'm going to do. But this one I'm confident of, my son is going to ly healed of this dreaded cancer. The Bible states that if I would walk upright before the Lord, pray in faith, believe, confess the Word daily, and demonstrate with my actions that I believe, surely my prayers will be answered. Certainly, if I followed this step-by-step approach to faith and prayer, everything would be alright. Undoubtedly, if I applied myself to the study and implementation of God's Word, surely my son would live. Surely!

I know to my family and friends that I appear to be perfectly valiant, courageous, and uncommonly resilient. I know that my tough exterior and composed disposition tell everyone that none of this bothers me. This facade, this rough appearance is nothing further from the truth. If you cut me, do I not bleed? Of course, I care. Of course, I worry. Of course, there is an overwhelming fear that, daily, attempts to overthrow and overshadow my duty and my responsibility toward the safety and well-being of my family. Contrary to popular belief, fear is not the opposite of faith. I believe in the Word of God with everything within me. Nonetheless, there are still bouts of anxiety and even doubt that we must wrestle with. No, the opposite of fear is love. And it is my love, for my family, and for my son, that compels me to continue making plans for a brighter tomorrow. With apprehensions, fears, questions, with unmet needs, my love for you says "keep going."

EVEN THE DARKEST NIGHT WILL END

Don't worry, don't be afraid. Although others may walk away, although others don't understand you, I will never leave you or abandon you; I will never loosen my grip on you, or leave you as an orphan. No matter what you face in this life, as long as there is breath in my lungs, I will be there for you Dontre', my son. There is one other person that keeps me committed. Crazy as it may sound, I have something to prove to my wife. Meaningless to others, but when you've experienced the ups and downs, the bends and curves, the hellfire and shame that we have, you realize the severity of your marital covenant and eventually begin taking it seriously. Getting married is more or less like enlisting in the military. It's easy to get married, but there will certainly be challenges in the marriage and you must remain in the marriage for the long haul and make it a success. So yes, I need to show my wife that she married the right man and that I am well equipped for the task at hand. Because we're in the rebuilding phase, I'm determined to do everything in my ability to foster confidence, hope, and adoration within our union. For this marriage to be fully restored, I'll have to give focused attention to my wife, treat her with tremendous consideration, express genuine gratitude, offer considerable support, and assure her that I will remain committed even during the most demanding moments.

I think one of the most incredible things in the world is to find somebody with whom you can develop a brilliantly profound and cheerfully stunning connection. And then, cultivate that relationship and watch it improve more and more as the years go by. Not all parents can, but I know that I have this kind of relationship with Dontre. Just like one piece of iron is used to sharpen another, our relationship as father and son has served to make both of us better. My years of experience and wisdom are being used to impart wisdom to his novice heart and mind. And his youthful immaturity and defiance have been used to toughen my extremely fragile patience and enlarge my appreciation for those around me. Dads and sons are two sides of the same coin; they complement each other in ways only God understands.

SEYMOND PERRY, SR.

On one hand, the father sees himself in his son. The father sees all of the promises, hopes, and dreams; he sees all of the dormant potentials that must be properly nurtured and cared for. On the other hand, the son sees the great conquering hero that he hopes to become. The son sees a man that is larger than life, that can make no mistakes, and is the very pinnacle of fatherhood and manhood in his eyes.

People with cancer are sometimes described as being brave, whether it's for going through treatment or coping with the emotional impact of a cancer diagnosis. I'm not quite sure that it's bravery as much as just trying to survive. Layoffs, financial worries, and illness can all create stress within a marriage. Worry, bitterness, and uncertainty can oftentimes bring out the most alarming characteristics in each party. And with strong negative feelings looming near, spouses usually make for easy and convenient targets to blame. Although we've never faced a challenge quite like this before, so far, the Perrys have been nothing short of brave, gallant, and daring. We have faced our health challenges even when we didn't understand or fully comprehend what was happening to us. That is not to say that we haven't had our fears, our doubts, or even worries. Fear is experienced by everyone. It triggers a natural survival instinct to fight or run and hide. But that's not what defines courage because bravery is acting in the face of fear, in the presence of doubt. Being heroic is facing what causes discomfort, hesitation, or doubt. Bravery is choosing to take a step forward, even when the statistics and the odds are stacked against you. We face a new episode, a new chapter.... together. Although we have faced so many obstacles in the past, our testimony and our confidence are unwavering. We are positive that we will come out triumphant. We use our past experiences and past victories as fuel for what we face today. From that dark past, from those hopeless situations, we have learned so many lessons. If our previous storms have taught us nothing else, they have taught us that even the darkest night will end and the sun will rise.

EVEN THE DARKEST NIGHT WILL END

"Seeds of faith are always within us; sometimes it takes a crisis to nourish and encourage their growth." — Susan Taylor

Chapter 2
Stand as a Soldier

B*e on guard; stand firm in your faith [in God, respecting His precepts and keeping your doctrine sound]. Act like [mature] men and be courageous; be strong* (1 Corinthians 16:13 AMP).

"The bravest are surely those who have the clearest vision of what is before them, glory and danger alike, and yet notwithstanding, go out to meet it." —Thucydides

I'd like to think of myself as being that heroic, confident, and daring soldier. But in all honesty, we have no idea how we will behave until we are confronted with the worst of our fears. Nonetheless, I do have a clear vision of the enemy that lies before us. My son, my junior, my posterity on the earth has been diagnosed with the dreadful disease known as cancer. Triumph and defeat stand before me as actual real possibilities. And what we see with our eyes, what we must endure and experience from day to day, makes it very grim and sometimes difficult to be courageous. To be honest, the easy thing to do would be to give up, to wave the white flag of surrender, that would be the smoothest course of action. There are moments when nervousness and dread are so overwhelming that you are paralyzed with panic and apprehension. You find yourself stuck somewhere between the proverbial rock and the hard place. Our current hard place is highly strenuous and makes it tricky and sometimes problematic to trigger one's faith. Because for the most part, we are living very active lives, at least as much as possible with Covid-19 still on an ever-increasing warpath. While others are battling a new aged pandemic, the Perrys are battling a foe that has been wandering the earth since 3,000 BC. People with cancer are

SEYMOND PERRY, SR.

oftentimes defined as fighting a battle (a war) with their fierce condition. And if this is true, at this junction in time, we (as a family) have only begun to fight. If we are at war, that would make us soldiers (new enlistees) but soldiers nonetheless. Young, old, middle-aged, inexperienced, and worn, regardless we are soldiers in a struggle against cancer. Whether we like it or not, this struggle (this skirmish) is to the death, the winner takes all (survival of the fittest). It will take all the strength we can muster and then some if we are to come out of this alive and intact. If we are to obtain total victory, it's going to take the fervor and power of the Eternal Spirit. "A clever general, therefore, avoids an army when its spirit is keen, but attacks it when it is sluggish and inclined to return" (The Art of War) If this strategy is correct, Satan has made a fatal flaw in attacking us now. Regardless of our dismal history, the Perry clan has only grown stronger and stronger with each passing battle. So, against all nervousness, against all doubt, and all anticipation, we have notably sustained and even increased our confidence in God's Word.

It is quite natural to experience feelings of worry, stress, and anxiety when faced with the threat of imminent danger. I believe adults experience this to an even greater degree because we have so many horrible life experiences to draw from. Satan only needs to whisper the smallest of problems within our ears and our imaginations will take that whisper and turn it into a world-breaking shout that leaves us crippled, hopeless, and residing within the lowest depths of despair. A child, on the other hand, typically only responds to what is in front of them, not what may or may not occur. My handsome son, Dontre', doesn't seem personally phased or troubled in the least by his recent diagnosis. He never utters a word of self-doubt, pity, remorse, or regret. We aren't sure whether it's childlike naivety or whether it's the power and faith of Jesus Christ within him. In the days, weeks, and months ahead, we would discover the source of this great tranquility and calm. Either way, there is a quite discernible and visible peace that overshadows him. We have spoken with Sean (his younger brother) and told him what the family is facing because of this crushing announcement. Sean is so very young (at least in my eyes), 2 years younger than Dontre'. Sean's personality and disposition are so much like mine. Once again, like father - like son. The Creator did such an amazing job of stamping all of my children with many of my physical, spiritual, and personality traits. Sean is so easygoing and unconcerned about everything around him. Sean, like his father, internalizes most circumstances, which makes it incredibly tricky to measure how he's really doing and what he's feeling. There are days that I feel like I'm neglecting Him because most of our focus has been centered around life's current disaster. Their sister, Sarai, is only a year old so she has no understanding of any of the troubles that we collectively face. She is just a baby and is simply happy to be alive. To our astonishment, her sweet innocence provides the family with cherished moments of relief from the drudgery of battling this disease. Sarah, my lovely wife, their mother, is fighting tooth and nail with ever-increasing belief in Jesus Christ. Understandably, she has been quite emotional at moments but she is developing and building herself up more and more every day. Because of the many doctor visits, and the countless trips back and forward, it can be mentally, physically, and so spiritually demanding. When home, she sleeps often. This places more of the day-to-day activities on my shoulders. And because of this, an added strain has been placed on the marriage relationship. Some would say catastrophe makes a marriage stronger, but first, catastrophe puts the marriage relationship to the test. And after all, we have gone through, we have survived in our marriage, another test is not what we want or desire.

    I'm a teacher by calling, anointing, and by occupation. One of the greatest pieces of advice I would give to any teacher is to always remain a student. Because of this, I've spent a lifetime acquiring information, wisdom, and knowledge. Some of this data has been collected through the revelation of the Holy Spirit. While like King Solomon, much of

SEYMOND PERRY, SR.

this wisdom has been acquired through agonizing trial and error. I have so many life-changing lessons on manhood and fatherhood, studies for relying on the invisible Jehovah-Shammah, and even reflections on fundamental humanity for my children. Many of these lessons were designed for a later and more mature time, especially for this child in particular. My God, he's only 13! With my human logic, I rationalize that he's not ready for many of these subjects, not just yet. As he grows older, as he matures, and is properly equipped (mentally, physically, and spiritually), I hoped to pass down all of this wisdom. Yet, some lessons were designed to be taught in phases, in stages. Each year capitalizing on the previous years' growth and progress. But the threat of death is on our doorsteps and we have no more time, at least not as much as I imagined. We are presently in a crucial confrontation, some would call this natural selection, and this will be on-the-field training. Whether he is ready or not, whether he is mature enough to handle them or not, as his father and spiritual leader, I must teach these complex lessons to Dontre' now. I must rely on the great Teacher to instruct me on how to properly educate him in this foreign way of thinking, this Kingdom way of thinking. Most importantly, Dontre' must receive, comprehend, and use each of these lessons now. Not tomorrow, not when he grows older, not when he feels like it. My son must fully embrace what I teach Him concerning the Word of Adonai and He must fully embrace what the Holy Spirit of Truth reveals to him personally. If the time to do what's right is always now, then Dontre' must act now!

I've been described as many things throughout my life. Nerd, arrogant, smart, and comical is a few that come to mind. The title that I wear proudly is Superman. If Superman was ever needed before, he was needed now. And operating like the Superman that I am, I jumped into action to save the day, to save my family, to save my son. There is an enemy that has attacked our home and threatens to utterly demolish one of our members. And whether it is right or wrong, I've taken the responsibility to save that member come hell or high water. Because our words are so important, I had already developed a confession of faith for myself. A confession of faith is a formal statement of Biblical beliefs. This confession is recited by an individual or group and is very similar to a creed. "One way to define wisdom is the ability to see into the future the consequences of your choices in the present. That ability can give you a completely different perspective on what the future might look like." (The Noticer: Andy Andrew - W. Publishing 2009). My confession was developed over several years and tailored specifically to the wants, needs, desires, and previous battles of my family. Because Dontre' was the person specifically under attack, he needed to have a personal confession to assist him through this painful journey. I used many portions of my confession to develop Dontre's individualized confession. At the outset of this trial, his confession was designed to be spoken daily. As time progressed, like pain medicine, he would need to recite it as often as needed. And it is through wisdom, the Spirit of Wisdom, that I was allowed to see that one of the biggest hurdles and obstacles to our success would be keeping Dontre' strong in faith. We must not ever fool ourselves or be lifted as false idols. Pain, suffering, torture, and spiritual wickedness will make the strongest of us crumble and cower in fear. If it were up to our enemy, Satan, we would deceive and control ourselves. But thanks be to Elohim who continually gives us victory. I've been approached on numerous occasions as to the validity of a confession. "Saying the word repeatedly does not make God move any faster in your life!" "God is going to do what He's going to do. No need for you to waste your time with pointless babble." "If it were that easy, all of us would have everything we said." I quickly and emphatically explain to these individuals that our confession is not for God; our confession is solely for our benefit. Several Scriptures promise justice and defense, His power and might towards the believer, and the Bread of Life's unmerited favor, and kindness towards His children. But there is a question that is posed: Will He find persistent, unwavering, heartfelt faith when He returns (Luke 18:8)? When He

SEYMOND PERRY, SR.

decides to move, will you be standing and operating from a place of trust and loyalty to His kingdom? Therefore, to keep our faith strong and consistent, we speak the Word of God strongly and consistently out of our mouths (Psalm 34:1). We speak firmly and with great boldness. We speak the Scriptures of old until the fire of God consumes everything that's not like Him. We recite, declare, and pronounce the Word of Yahweh until everything within us and within our lives looks and functions as His Word promised.

Taking the Lord at His Word, knowing that He cannot lie, we rallied to our son's side and taught him how to stand in faith for manifested healing. That does not mean that it was simple or easy, or that the process was straightforward or without challenges. Our family is a very musically inclined family. From singing to instruments, we love music in all of its many forms. There is one particularly strenuous moment that comes to mind, it must have been a Wednesday night. The family prepared to leave home to attend Praise Team practice. Whether he lacked physical strength or was just not feeling well, Dontre' decided to remain at home. Practices typically last anywhere from one and a half to two hours. During practice, Dontre' began to repeatedly text his mother that he was in unbearable pain and not feeling well at all. Sarah instructed him to take his pain medication and that we would be home as quickly as possible. We concluded rehearsal soon thereafter and quickly came home to attend to his needs. When we arrived home, we found him grimacing in pain, sobbing through uncontrollable tears. Like any caring mother, Sarah asked if he wanted to go to the hospital; his response was no. Partly because a hospital visit is never quick and easy. Hospital stays were typically a minimum of three days, three days of complete upheaval for the entire family. If Dontre' is in the hospital, mom must be there with him. If mom is there, dad must take on all of the duties of transporting children, preparing meals, day to day household chores, and this does not include still having a very young career in teaching. Because he did not want

EVEN THE DARKEST NIGHT WILL END

to be admitted to the hospital, I instructed Dontre' to sit at the table while I began washing dishes. I instructed him to recite his confession of faith. With some strong encouragement from dad, with tears in his eyes, my brave son obeyed and recited his confession. Because the symptoms and discomfort persisted, I instructed him to repeat his confession. with a little reluctance but still in obedience, Dontre' obeyed his father and said his confession of faith. "How do you feel son?" He tells me that he's still hurting and still in a lot of pain. But from his tone of voice and the dried tears, I can tell that his symptoms are much better. This issue is, I don't think he yet realizes that his symptoms are subsiding. For a third time, I ask him to declare his confession once more, and as before, he reads his confession. But this time even to my amazement, there is more confidence, more passion, and more power that carries every word off his lips. I know this power all too well; this is the strength of the Breath of The Almighty. And although I have experienced it often, it is something to see the power of God upon your child. At that moment, it reassures me that all of the lessons and all the teachings are working. Once he concludes speaking, I ask, "How do you feel?" Dontre's response: "I feel great." It's one thing to teach a person a lesson. It's something altogether different for them to apply what you have taught them and for them are that it works. And just like most lessons, some are best learned through experience. I lovingly kiss him on the forehead goodnight and tell him to get some much-needed rest.

Being diagnosed with any illness, especially a long-term health condition, can be frightening and almost debilitating. Once you move past the initial shock and horror, you still have to cope with the daily stresses of this horrific battle. This specific encounter was only one of many episodes that we would face on a pretty regular basis. Countless days were spent in agonizing discomfort, in freezing hospital rooms, and in lonesome doctor's visits. Numerous nights were spent pacing the floors of our home, intensely praying over the family and speaking

SEYMOND PERRY, SR.

directly to our sworn enemy. But time and time again, we would valiantly overcome each attack; we would always overcome together as a family (Revelation 12:11). Through it all, we taught Dontre how to confess the Word of Jehovah over his own body and trust the Spirit of Counsel to manifest the results. It was important to teach our son how to use his faith. Although we are his parents, although we can stand in the gap and intercede on his behalf, in the end, he would have to stand in faith for himself. And as the days, weeks, and months progressed, we saw Dontre's and the entire family's convictions increase by leaps and bounds. Even so, everyone is prone to the ravishing effects of stress. Although you keep winning the day-to-day battles, there is always the threat of tomorrow, and that threat (real or not) brings about stress. This stress, this disease, can make anyone susceptible to demonic attack. So, as we tackle the stresses of cancer, the stresses of marriage, and the stresses of parenting, we must also handle and manage the everyday stresses of just being a human being.

In most healthy situations, a dad is a hero his son hopes to be, this we know to be true. From the way they walk to the way they talk, from the way they brush their teeth to their odd sense of humor, the apple doesn't fall too far from the tree. Before the comic books and cartoons, before the strength of professional athletes and the mesmerizing charm of Broadway, a father was a son's very first champion. And with every ounce of my being, like the knight in shining armor, I am determined to valiantly and courageously save the day. It is not pride or arrogance that fuels this attitude of triumph; it is not blind faith or even foolish naivety. No, it is something much greater and much stronger than arrogance, foolishness, haughtiness, or stupidity. It is my love that grants me the ability to keep moving forward; against all odds, against all logic and reason, the love I have for my family is what keeps me calm and resolved during these treacherous moments. German social psychologist, Erich Fromm certainly knew something about unreliable times. Fromm wrote, "Love is an act of faith, and whoever is of little

EVEN THE DARKEST NIGHT WILL END

faith is also of little love." And since I am a man of much faith, I am also a man of much love.

Amid this, the strength and weaknesses, the joy and the tears, we continued to remain in faith. And even to our amazement, we have maintained our hope and trust in the Lord. But what's the alternative, to admit defeat, to feel shame, and to wallow in regret, God forbid? But even with the faith of Abraham, on October 17, 2020, we are once again haunted by another extended hospital stay. Dontre' had been experiencing some very troublesome complications for about a week. The doctors were expecting him to be admitted to the hospital for two to three weeks. Once again, against all the odds, on October 24, 2020, he and Sarah returned home. In our very midst, the Lord is working a miracle in my family. He is answering prayers and showing Himself strong on behalf of His people. No matter the challenge or the obstacle, our resolve in Elohim could not be shaken. He continues to perform miracles right before our eyes and we continue to celebrate and share the testimony of His goodness. Those around us would oftentimes comment how much they were amazed at our resolve, our growth, and our tenacity. Many times, they would attempt to applaud us and what we were doing but we were very conscious to direct the honor back to the Lord and His never-failing promises. It is the Lord Himself who promises that even the darkest night will end and the sun will rise.

"Feed your faith, and your fears will starve to death." — Unknown

Chapter 3
I Always Win

They will fight against you, but they will not [ultimately] prevail over you, for I am with you [always] to protect you and deliver you," says the Lord (Jeremiah 1:19 AMP).

To grow in knowledge, you must be placed in circumstances where you don't know. To grow in strength, you must be placed within environments where you are weak. To grow in patience, you must be placed in situations that require you to wait. David, the man that shared the same desires as God, poetically writes in the Psalms "*I waited patiently for the Lord*". "God never promises that He will immediately wave His magic wand and deliver us from the pit. On the contrary, David conveys the sense that his rescue, while certain, was a long time in coming." (Rich Wagner) So often, when you are in the depths of an ordeal, time seems to be altered. What seems to be a lengthy period for us, in reality, is but a brief moment. The saying goes "time flies when you're having fun." If this is true, time must stand still for those who are suffering. When we are faced with split-second decisions, life or death choices, those few moments seem to linger for a lifetime. Our battle with the gruesome titan known as cancer was no different. People who live with and beyond cancer are often described as survivors. It's a very common term and is used by some cancer charities as well as people who've endured the ravages of cancer. Anyone that has seen the devastation that any type of cancer causes knows just why you're thought of as a survivor. The individual is literally in a fight for their life; a life that is so full of promises and uncertainty. Within any crisis are moments of vast danger and uncertainty. For anyone to thrive

SEYMOND PERRY, SR.

during a catastrophe, they need to have a renewed mind and a change of heart. This paradigm shift must take place for the unknown risks that lie ahead and to help minimize unforeseen damage and injury. Is this an easy process? No, this process is heavy beyond any doubt. Is this a quick process? How long it takes a person to have a change of mind is completely up to the individual. How does one make this kind of change? You make this sort of adjustment by bringing your wants, needs, and desires to a bare minimum. Lowering your day-to-day requirements will aid you in remaining focused on the stuff that's truly necessary for life. While there, you constantly evaluate and reevaluate your current situation in case you need to quickly adjust your strategy. And after checking and rechecking, developing several contingency plans, and even further developing your skills and knowledge, you still feel unprepared and at a loss. Because even if you defeat this monster, you will be forever changed (mentally, physically, and spiritually). The reality forever haunts you that this demon may rear its ugly head once again in your life. So many people survive the initial blow of cancer only to succumb to its covert operations years later. That's a scary thought, to save someone today just so they can die tomorrow.

    Made up of gray fats and proteins, the human brain is astonishing. It is one of the most complex systems known to mankind. From this three-pound clump of matter, we can give life to art, sports, personality, and morals. Even with all of these intricacies, the human mind is only capable of actively focusing on one idea at a time. American pastor, Joel Osteen, teaches that you cannot expect victory and plan for defeat. If someone were "double-minded" like this, it would suggest that they do not expect victory at all. And in our minds, victory, success, and triumph were inevitable. We did not know exactly when the total healing would manifest but we did know healing was unavoidable. If our hands and hearts remained pure and clean before the Lord, and wholeheartedly obeyed the voice of the Holy Spirit, we have been promised an assured and expected end. And although we wait with

EVEN THE DARKEST NIGHT WILL END

great patience, we do not perform it passively. Waiting on the Lord is not like waiting at the corner for the bus. Waiting on the Lord is not like waiting for the thunderstorm to cease. Waiting on the Lord is not like waiting for a beautiful sunrise. Waiting on the Lord is an active waiting where we live each present moment to the fullest. In doing so you will discover there are signs of the One you are waiting for. When actively waiting on the Lord you will discover that He was there in the fire with you the entire time. But after that ye have suffered a while, the Lord will make you perfect, establish, strengthen, settle you (1 Peter 5:10 KJV). Then you will have the testimony of King David: our focus and attention are on the Lord our God until He has mercy on us (Psalm 123:2). It was in January of 2021 that our faith was remarkably satisfied with the most astounding news. It was a regularly scheduled follow-up and with the help and grace of El Shaddai, Dontre' is making remarkable progress. After several screenings and tests, this follow-up doctor's visit shows that all cancer has vacated Dontre's body. He has been declared cancer free! Receiving good news can be just as overwhelming as receiving bad news. Sometimes hearing that you've got something that you wanted so desperately can range from total relief to actual anxiety, because you wonder if it will be long-lasting. And the human in us wants good news to follow up by even greater news. But as to not be greedy or ungrateful, we must take time to thank the Father for the "big" and the perceived "small" answered prayers. I cannot fully articulate just how joyous and excited our family was during this period. "We made it!" "We did what the Lord said and it worked." "Above all odds, we know the Lord to be faithful to His Word." Everyone around us was in awe of our loyalty and trust in our heavenly Father. Probably because had to actually walk out of this process, we were not amazed at all. It's what we knew He would do all along. We knew He would do it because faith is now; the Word of God is forever established and settled in heaven; faith says it's already done. This is what we confessed daily. This is what we prayed daily. This is

SEYMOND PERRY, SR.

what we stood in unwavering agreement for daily. This is the moment we knew the power of Yahweh could and would produce. With this breaking news, the worst is definitely behind us as we triumphantly rejoice in the favorable report that has been presented to us. Although he is cancer free, we must still stay the course with his prescribed medical treatments. Dontre' still has to finish one last cycle of chemotherapy, but once this cycle is over, the nightmare will be over and we will be free to have our lives back.

A believer in the Lord Jesus Christ does not need to ever be defeated by anything or anyone. Why? Because the life-giving power of the Everlasting Father and the chain-breaking power of the Holy Ghost can allow you to avoid and overcome any defeat. When we are convinced beyond all doubt that Jehovah loves us and that He loves our family, we have little issue believing that we will ultimately be victorious. At times, we seemingly have just enough to get by. It would do us well to focus on the fact that we are still getting by. The Lord has not failed to provide for us and He never will. This is not to downplay or minimize the circumstances of life. Life can be extremely overwhelming. But it is the will of God that all of His children be victorious; He built us to be overcomers! Since my days of playing football until now, I have never been one to quietly accept defeat; I hate losing at anything. Once while my wife and I were dating, I remember her beating me at a video game. The date was instantly ruined and the evening was now a complete loss. Why? All because I was extremely resentful that I lost. My pride was crushed because the girl I'm trying to impress had bested me in a task I'm supposed to be good at. I don't care if it's Monopoly, weight lifting, or cleaning the house, I goal and aim to be the best and to never lose. Fortunately for me, most of my life I've been on the victor's side. I don't know whether I'm right or wrong but for me, it's the only way to live. I enter most situations expecting to win and when I don't win, it can be almost unbearable to endure the barrage of emotions that come my way. So, in most instances, I do whatever it takes (within the rules of course) to come out ahead. Like the great Vince Lombardi shouted: "winning isn't everything. It's the only thing."

Even when someone experiences triumph, the never-ending battles of life can still leave us feeling beat down, dejected, and confused. These conflicts can make you feel as if you're still a total loser. Why do I have to keep facing these troubles? Just because we are facing a difficult season, we begin to think we're doing a horrible job of managing ourselves and steering our lives. And more times than not, you falsely think you're the only one who feels like this. Maybe today, at this moment, you don't feel like much of a champion. It's possible that you've gone through some battles and you feel like you've lost. But the Word of God declares that you are victorious! But, how can you be a winner when you feel like such a loser? How can you focus on overcoming the world when you can't even "shoot a fish in a barrel." You feel the crushing disappointment of wrong choices and blundered decisions. We've all pointed the finger of blame at ourselves when the truth is some things just cannot be avoided. Everyone has beaten themselves up for not performing as well as they thought they should. Nonetheless, with all of those feelings and emotions raging, the Word of Jehovah still declares that you're a winner. It doesn't matter how you feel. We do not base our decisions or our belief system on feelings. It doesn't matter what battles you think you have lost. When it's all said and done, God will make you victorious over this world and its evil system. Come what may, the battles or the enemy, we have been declared winners. The Bible assures us that the Master and His Son are Victors and that we are heirs of that same victory (1 Corinthians 15:57).

Because of our newly pronounced victory, there is now a huge sigh of relief expressed by all. A heavy burden that has been lifted from the backs of my family. We are so overjoyed that we are beginning to make plans for family trips, parties, and celebrations that commemorate this

SEYMOND PERRY, SR.

momentous occasion. My son is now cancer free! Our blood family, our church family, and as far as we know, the entire world have joined together in celebrating my son's new lease on life. So, with great joy in our hearts, we continue with the regimen of chemotherapy as prescribed by the medical staff. This means we still have to make the 45-minute drives for treatments. This still means the chemo bags. This still means the occasional loss of appetite. Nonetheless, we are headed toward the end of this crisis. The snowfall of February 14, 2021, made this trip extremely slow and challenging. As was our custom, Sarah and I came to church on that Sunday. By the time church had ended, it had begun to snow and the forecast showed that it would only continue for the next several days. I knew Sarah was exhausted because she had been with Dontre' over the previous three days. We feared that if we didn't pick Dontre up today that he would be stuck at the hospital for the next several days, or at least until all of the snow cleared. I instructed her to stay home, get some rest and I would travel to Little Rock to retrieve Dontre'. I texted several of the men in the church so they could be praying for us as we traveled to and from the hospital. When his treatment was finished, we faced a slight dilemma. People who are receiving treatment for cancer are often very sensitive to extreme temperatures. Exposure to these extreme temperatures can send their bodies into a very debilitating pain crisis. Like an Eskimo in the wilderness of Alaska, I wrapped him up with all I had and rushed him to our car. From there, we slowly and carefully navigated the 45-minute trip back home. Regardless of the weather, despite the tremendous exhaustion in our bodies, we were filled with wonderful joy and bliss because of the ultimate success provided to us through the True Vine.

 A renowned advocate of nonviolent resistance, Mahatma Gandhi understood all too well how hardships, setbacks, and victory affect the human spirit. He was quoted as saying: "When I despair, I remember that all through history the way of truth and love have always won. There have been tyrants and murderers, and for a time, they can seem invincible, but in the end, they always fall. Think of it - always." No matter how big or how bad the enemy may be, they all fall. And this day, the Perrys raise the victory flag against the dreaded tyrant known as cancer. Though we would rather not have experienced any of this, I can say that we are better because of it. Cancer exposed the extreme magnitude, profound seriousness, and all-in-composing scope of my passion and devotion to my family. As much as everyone desires it, love is one of the great mysteries of life. Most individuals' first encounter with love is at birth, received from a mother who is relieved but also very afraid. As time progresses, our affection for family and friends only grows stronger. As we discover music, sports, art, and the beauty of nature, we learn that love extends to every facet of life. Poets attempt to capture its essence with words, musicians write heartfelt songs conveying the joys and pains of it. Actors convincingly portray it for others to see, while preachers tirelessly teach about it expecting the world to be a better place. From inception to the grave, all of humanity is in desperate pursuit of love. And "the moment you have in your heart this extraordinary thing called love and feel the depth, the delight, the ecstasy of it, you will discover that for you the world is transformed." -Jiddu Krishnamurti After cancer, that's just what the world is for me, different. Not in a bad way, not necessarily in a good way; the world is just different. On second thought, maybe the world isn't different; I believe I just have a transformed perspective from which I view it. Whether the world is different or I see differently, what I can say is life is different after experiencing cancer.

Money, independence, a sense of community, and many more are reasons adults feel compelled to find gainful employment, to find a job. For the most part, grown-ups obtain jobs because they have financial and household obligations. But adventure and excitement give cheerful meaning and concentrated purpose to life. In our contemporary society, we don't encounter hair-raising adventures in our day-to-day affairs. There are no dreary castles to storm; there are no savage

SEYMOND PERRY, SR.

civilizations to conquer utterly. With the advancement in modern technology, there is little need to chop trees for firewood; there is little need to collect water from the creek. Despite this, I have been afforded this grand adventure and my brave son is at my side to keep me company. Father and son fight the blinding snow and deceptive ice in tandem. Although we never spoke about it or discussed it, I know both of us were secretly enjoying this exciting experience; this remarkable event would soon become a lasting memory engraved within our hearts and minds. As we traveled down the dark highway toward home, in my vivid imagination, I was the fearless knight in shimmering armor, setting out to retrieve his captured loved one. Setting out to save his son. And now that the mysterious and lethal dragon called cancer has been utterly and completely slain, we can safely return to our glorious castle lodged securely within the emerald mountains. Every hostile attacker that has come against us, we have overcome. With lacerations, serious bruises, and even missing limbs, we have beat the statistics and made it victoriously to the other side. We made it while frightened, terrified, and frequently in tears; regardless, we made it as a family; we made it together. Our family's various crusades and misadventures prove that even the darkest night will end and the sun will rise.

"FOR EVERY MOUNTAIN, there is a miracle." — Robert H. Schuller

Chapter 4
The Lernaean Hydra

We are pressured in every way [hedged in], but not crushed; perplexed [unsure of finding a way out], but not driven to despair; [9] *hunted down and persecuted, but not deserted [to stand alone]; struck down, but never destroyed;* [10] *always carrying around in the body the dying of Jesus, so that the [resurrection] life of Jesus also may be shown in our body* (2 Corinthians 4:8 - 10 AMP).

"Men are practical creatures; we are doers, task-driven. But that doesn't mean that we grow by reading only concepts and principles. We also want to be inspired. We need to grab hold of something larger than ourselves." - The Expeditionary Man: Rich Wagner.

And no matter how special I believe myself to be, I am no different than any other man. At least in this regard, we long for a thrilling adventure; we crave an inspiring encounter of some sort. If you would survey a thousand men, I'm sure most, if not all, would agree that they want to feel alive. Certainly, the Lord of hosts answered my prayers and gave me an experience of a lifetime. Probably not the way I was expecting or ever imagined, but one thing was for sure, I felt alive. My son having cancer was a great challenge and an awe-inspiring exploit. This was a daunting task but it was a challenge that I was eager and more than willing to undertake. Some of my reasons may have been a bit selfish: to prove that I'm a good leader, to prove that I'm the hero that I claim to be, to prove that I can be trusted with the lives of those around me. On a more righteous note, I also want to demonstrate to the world that our God is real. Of all the motives I possess, the latter

SEYMOND PERRY, SR.

is probably the noblest and godly of reasons. Above all else, my heart desires to show a faithless society that these Bible stories are not just stories but they occurred in history. These ancient events of old All of mankind need to know that the Redeemer of the Bible is alive and on His throne. If for no other reason, the life of our son gives evidence of this. Jehovah Nissi, in all of His greatness and splendor, has performed the impossible in our lives; He has healed our son of cancer. Because of this astonishing revelation, anyone who hears our story should be inspired to believe in this amazing God. I pray that those who view my family will be able to see our Lord and Savior. People have varying rationales as to why they feel the need to prove themselves to others. One person may be motivated because they feel as if they've been wronged or unappreciated. Other individuals know their value and worth but have been dismissed time and time again. Because of this, they want to make a statement that shows others the error of their ways. Whatever the case may be, proving your point is oftentimes seen as the only way to rise above and transform into something beautiful and new. Although beyond difficult and taxing, this was the moment and the situation of a lifetime for me to prove all those aspirations, dreams, and goals to everyone.

Hercules, of Greek mythology, was a man who was a definite thing to prove. On his second labor, Hercules was to kill the Lernaean Hydra. The dreaded Lernaean Hydra is a furious beast of antiquity. More often known simply as the Hydra, it is a winding water monster in Greek and Roman mythology. From the murky waters of the swamps, the Hydra would ascend to terrorize and oppress the countryside. Of its many features, the Hydra had poisonous breath and poisonous blood so fatal that even its scent was deadly. The Hydra had many heads that possessed a regeneration feature: for every head chopped off, the Hydra would regrow two heads. This gruesome beast was not easy prey because one of the heads was immortal and therefore very indestructible. In the orthodox Hydra myth, the monster is eventually

EVEN THE DARKEST NIGHT WILL END

killed by Hercules when he acquired the assistance of his nephew Lolaus to cut off all of the monster's heads and burn the neck using a sword and fire. The more I think about this deadly monster named the Hydra, the more I begin to relate its monstrosity to that of cancer. We have won, but there is a part of me that is still afraid. Afraid that in time, one month, one year, ten years, the head of cancer will grow back. After treatment ends, one of the most common concerns for a survivor is that cancer will come back. Dontre' never spoke of his fears, dread, or even what he was worried about. But as his father and protector, I am surely concerned about a cancer recurrence. Try as I might to not dwell on these possibilities, deep within, I know this to be a very real possibility. Try as I might be testone-faced, I'm a normal human with normal feelings and emotions, and having a fear of recurrence is very normal.

Aren't soldiers allowed to be afraid? Aren't soldiers allowed to have questions and doubts? Although he ultimately won the battle, I'm sure at some point Hercules was afraid. Although I stand as a soldier of the Lord Jesus Christ, I still have concerns. Other than our Wonderful Counselor, I'm afraid I can't share with anyone. You would think I'd have a much different disposition seeing that we are currently standing in victory. As much as I've trained my mind to be a deadly weapon, there are days I feel my mind is working against me. Currently, we're living on the outskirts of the "Promised Land", but my brain won't stop focusing on all the bad things that could happen. As long as we've been married, the good times never last all that long. So now, I live expecting something bad, dreadful, or seriously disastrous is going to occur. My son has just been declared cancer free but I can't shake these emotions, this anxiety. Try as I might to put on a brave face and shield my true concerns from the world, deep inside I know and surely the Father knows the truth. But as all great warriors do, suppress these things called feelings and keep moving forward. With the many uncertainties I have about tomorrow, I continue to stand against everything that

SEYMOND PERRY, SR.

would come to steal, kill, or destroy my family and my lineage. I fight against the tricks and plots of our sworn enemy. I stand firm with the shield of faith as protection against the fiery darts that would attack and overtake my mind. Most importantly, we use our only offensive weapon, the Sword of the Spirit (which is the Word of God). We have used this Sword to cut off the heads of the cancerous Hydra that plagues our son's life. We will not cease; we will not rest. We will be relentless in our efforts; we will not give up until the beast is utterly defeated. As a husband and a father, I have been uniquely prepared to serve and defend my family. And over the years, I've discovered that there is so much more to guarding my household than merely being physically powerful. There is so much more to protecting my family than taking the typical bullet in place of my wife and children. There comes a moment when a man must offer his life (physical and spiritual) for the benefit of my family.

It was just January that we waved the banner of victory. Triumph after wonderful triumph, celebration after glorious celebration, we slowly began to enjoy our lives again. Making plans for summer vacation and even the upcoming school year, we were doing our best to put this dreaded nightmare behind us. We even enjoyed the opportunity to celebrate Dontre's fourteenth birthday. Although we tried our best not to accept it, bit by bit the symptoms of cancer returned. Spelled out in big bold letters, we saw all the writing on the wall. Much like the mythological creature, though you cut one cancerous head off, several grow back in its place. After more treatments and more oxygen, the doctors confirm that the cancer has returned. To our horror and dismay, by the end of March horrific cancer began to rapidly spread again. We had won once; we can win again. If there is nothing too hard for God, then there is nothing too hard for the Perry family. Like the old negro spiritual: "We shall overcome"! So once again, we suit for another daring campaign. Unlike those who become hopeless and discouraged, we find the wherewithal

EVEN THE DARKEST NIGHT WILL END

to maintain our faith in Jehovah. Armed with the strength of heaven, we again transition from hospital stay to hospital stay. We slash and cut and claw our way back to our rightful place of victory. Try as we might, through our prayers, our fasting, even our tears, the hideous horror is more powerful than before; it has grown two heads in the place of one. And much to everyone's regret, it is moving stronger and harder than before. As much as friends and loved ones try to encourage us individually and collectively, we can't help but feel that there is something we did wrong, that somehow this recent development is our fault. Did we miss or overlook something? Did we not pray the right prayer or say the correct Scriptures? Was our faith not strong enough to overcome the day of adversity (Proverbs 24:10)? Did we celebrate too soon? Is it possible that we have not been in faith this entire time? Do I still have enough fight left in me to engage in combat once again? As all of these questions and emotions swirl through our heads, we must find a way to strengthen, fortify, and rebuild our resolve in Christ. Because Dontre' has been hospitalized for much longer than usual, Sarah has not been home. If she hasn't been home, this means the other two children are with me. During the day, Sean goes to school but Sarai is not old enough to attend school just yet and this poses a dilemma for me. You can't bring a two-year-old into a high school classroom during a global pandemic. On April 5, 2021, I notified my job that Dontre' had been admitted to the hospital with a collapsed lung. As much of a provider as I am, I do know where my priorities lay. As much as it hurt to inform them, after spending the past few years building this career, I notified them that I would not be returning to work until I could get childcare situated. I must, for my family, remain fully engaged in this physical and spiritual warfare. For the sake of my family, I must find a way to keep going. For my posterity on the earth, there must be a way for us to make it through this season of utter darkness. For my son, we must find a way to win. I am not willing to pay the price of defeat; therefore, I am determined to win. I refuse to lose!

SEYMOND PERRY, SR.

I am taken by surprise when I realize that there is something within me shifting, gradually changing, and it's not for the better. This thing that is ever so subtly changing is for the worse. I've spent years training my senses, honing my intellect, and strengthening my spirit. Usually, I can quickly detect when something is out of place, especially when that object lies within me. I can't explain or even fully describe exactly what's wrong but I know when something isn't quite right. German philosopher, Friedrich Nietzsche, had this to say about battling monsters: "Whoever fights monsters should see to it that in the process he does not become a monster." And just maybe that's what I'm experiencing, could it be that I am slowly transforming into a monster as I fight the monster called cancer? Try as I might to maintain my humanity, try as I might to retain my godliness, there are parts of me, my character, my personality, that are becoming very grotesque and very unattractive. When we survey someone's life in totality, a history of trauma seems to be the greatest indicator of this appalling transformation. Oftentimes we discover that the most hideous serial killer was seriously and severely abused in childhood. On the other hand, the catalyst for becoming a monster was generally a complete failure from societal support. And usually, with the smallest of nudges, the person begins a vicious cycle in which they become a vicious predator. To my amazement, with all of the advancements in technology, with all of the recent discoveries in space, and even with the newest spiritual revelations, monsters continue to saturate the lives of humanity. Monsters of nuclear destruction, freak climate changes, giants of treachery, we are even fearful of foreign villains. And some of us, like little children, are afraid of the things that go bump in the night. People may lie to themselves and they may never admit it to anyone else, but it is very difficult to survive in this world without becoming a monster. You're either devoured by a monster or you inevitably become one out of a great necessity to survive. There are varying types of creatures and monsters. There are your everyday run-of-the-mill

EVEN THE DARKEST NIGHT WILL END

enemies and then there are actual monsters. Normally, monsters are huge in stature and incredibly destructive. But no matter the shape or size, no matter the geographical location, no matter the race or cultural background, all monsters have one main purpose for existence: DESTRUCTION!

So, we continue to battle the internal and the external demons, we continue to battle the physical and the spiritual demons. We continue to fight with the only real weapon we have, the Word of the Eternal Judge (Ephesians 6:17). Whoever said "experience is the best teacher," must have been faced with some of life's most extreme challenges, and they must have learned some very valuable lessons as well. If you have ever attempted to learn a topic simply by reading a book, you may have realized it wasn't easy at all. People often forget that trying new things ourselves is usually the best and most profound way of learning. Real-world experience is typically the best teacher because it's hands-on and deals directly with our five senses. Unknown to me, the class was in session and the Master Teacher was cultivating within me some serious truths. One such lesson was to "watch and pray." To state it simply, we pray according to the Word of God. Your adversary, the Devil, will make alterations to his ways of attack based on your prayers. You must be mindful (watchful) of these adjustments as they manifest and modify your methods and strategies of prayer as well. Many believers are defeated due to their relaxed prayer life. The Christian is playing checkers while Satan is playing chess. Completely different from those of the past, this strike was so unexpected and so swift that we had very little time to take countermeasures. Although I secretly feared this would occur, when I actually saw it, I faced great difficulty in actually regaining my bearings. The Mighty One's Word teaches us to not be ignorant of our opposition's schemes. God's Word teaches us to always be alert, to be clear-minded, and to pray accordingly. Covered by the grace of the Almighty, on April 10, 2021, the Spirit of God directed me to develop a new Confession of Faith. This confession would address

SEYMOND PERRY, SR.

the new methods of attack, areas of faith we felt were lacking, and reinforce areas that were already strong. Again, this confession is not to prompt the Lord to move or to coerce the Lord into action. Our proclamation is designed to keep our faith sturdy and anchored in His Word. Keeping our belief system resilient serves two main purposes: 1) we can only please the Lord through faith, and 2) when the Breath of The Almighty moves we want Him to find us operating in faith (Luke 18:8). With new fire and tenacity in our hearts, we declare the Word of our Deliverer over ourselves, over our family, over this terrible situation. Knowing and trusting that the perfect will of God will be performed in our lives and in our children's lives.

Dads share their hard-earned wisdom with their children for several reasons. To make their children's lives better, to help them forego some of the pitfalls and mistakes they've made, fathers pour into their children to ensure future generations are blessed by their knowledge. Various fathers possess various justifications as to why they impart so much information to their children, especially their sons. Nonetheless, we have arrived at this junction in life, and my hopes, the great aspirations that I have for my son, are being threatened. Everyone has witnessed an adult drag a screaming kid from the store and something just doesn't feel right. Does this child belong to this adult? Most people have seen an altercation between an adult and a child that was just a little too rough. Was this a recurring episode or was this merely an accident? Is the frightened little girl in the backseat of a passing car being abducted or is she legitimately afraid of something else? In all of these situations, there could be a bad guy or you could be overreacting. But my plight is so different, my child is being threatened and I have no physical person to direct my frustrations towards. There is no 1-800 hotline that will accept my detailed report of the perpetrator. No law enforcement unit can arrest the bad guy and rescue my son. Right now, we feel deceived, let down, and very much disappointed and in the same breath I am more resolved in my efforts

EVEN THE DARKEST NIGHT WILL END

than ever. If we have to walk this lonesome road thousand times over, I will do it to see victory; I will do it to behold my son happy and healthy. In some ways, this may be nothing more than self-seeking devotion and some sort of macho bravado. In some ways, this could be me, myself, and I that is providing the strength to carry on. But as time progresses, if a person was to lay it all on the line, you quickly realize that it must be something or Someone altogether different that is compelling him to carry on. Because in my natural human power, I wanted to give up a long time ago. From kids to marriage, from jobs to ministry, I've wanted to quit all of them at one time or another. Nonetheless, we are still here, standing strong and committed. And there is only one force this strong, this powerful, this absolute. There is only one power so intense as to move mountains and calm the storms of life. There is only one force that is powerful enough to conquer death and the grave; that force is the power of love.

"My love for you has no depth, its boundaries are ever-expanding. My love and my life with you will be a never-ending story. My love with you is never-ending" -M. Christina White

And it is my never-ending love for Dontre' that encourages and motivates me to carry on. Against all logic, against all reason, love is the rationale behind our every decision.

Godzilla, The Blob, Vampires and Werewolves, King Kong, and even the Grendel are all monsters that represent many of mankind's deepest, darkest, and most disturbing fears. These bizarre demons, including the Hydra, mirror many of the power dynamics, biases, and worries of communities and the individuals in them. Hypertrichosis, also known as "werewolf disease," is a condition of excessive hair growth throughout the body. A rare disease called erythropoietic protoporphyria (EPP) is known to exhibit several symptoms similar to that of the fabled vampire. And the list goes on and on of how we have taken our ailments and given them a life of their own. Diseases, a lot like monsters, oftentimes cripple our hearts and minds from making

SEYMOND PERRY, SR.

any forward progress. But I will not be stopped, I will not give in and I absolutely will not surrender. If I must sever the head of cancer over and over again, I will do it. With love in my heart and the Word of God as my only weapon, I will be victorious. All dreaded creatures have a weakness, an Akilies heel; I must simply locate cancer's weakness and strike. Although Greek mythology and Hollywood movies may be fictional, they do point us in a most hopeful direction. No matter how strong, menacing, gruesome, or destructive, the enemy, the villain, the hideous creature is always defeated. The hero always wins; the captives are always set free. No matter the size of the hideous foe, despite the devastation and destruction, even the darkest night will end and the sun will rise.

EVEN THE DARKEST NIGHT WILL END

"When we long for life without difficulties, remind us that oaks grow strong in contrary winds, and diamonds are made under pressure." — Peter Marshall

Chapter 5
Lay Down Your Life

No one has greater love [nor stronger commitment] than to lay down his own life for his friends (John 15:13 AMP).

"Real love is unconditional and should be evident in all love relationships (1 Corinthians 13:4 - 7).

The foundation of a solid relationship with your child is unconditional love. Only that type of love relationship can assure a child's growth to his total potential. Only this foundation of unconditional love can assure prevention of problems such as feelings of resentment, being unloved, guilt, fear, insecurity." (How to really love your child - Dr. Ross Campbell). Over the years, I have struggled with being a good husband but I love my children. That is not to say I don't love my wife; I've just found it "easier" to love my children (for whatever reason). I can proudly declare that I love them under all conditions. I have three children (two boys and a girl) and they are each so very unique, both in body and mind. The love I possess for them constantly and simultaneously consists of distress, terror, pride, joy, laughter, sorrow, rage, disappointment, and anguish. But when you say that you are willing to die for a loved one, you never truly believe that you will ever have to do it. Thomas Paine tells us "These are the times that try men's souls; the summer soldier and the sunshine patriot will, in this crisis, shrink from the service of his country; but he that stands it now, deserves the love and thanks of man and woman. Tyranny, like hell, is not easily conquered; yet we have this consolation with us, that the harder the conflict, the more glorious the triumph." I would say these are the times where "the rubber meets the road". It was G. Michael

SEYMOND PERRY, SR.

Hopf who said, "Hard times create strong men, strong men create good times, good times create weak men, and weak men create hard times." All of us have reached a junction in life where our fortitude is put on trial. Being a powerful man is a choice and a discipline; it is not a natural quality that is given to the few and the fortunate. Whatever the challenge, a person must choose to be strong, obtain a new perspective and make decisive actions to thrive. I do feel all of my life's difficulties were orchestrated to mold me into a tougher man because my life has been full of many moments of difficulty. At least in my mind, that's what I presumed.

"The idea of a man taking responsibility for his family's spiritual, physical, and emotional needs is biblical, honorable, and loving. But I am convinced that it is also over-glorified by the church today. The far more pressing issue is the tendency of fathers to pay so much attention to material needs that they overlook a family's spiritual needs." —Rich Wagner

Especially while a young parent, I was very guilty of this grievous mistake. Partly because of my upbringing, my parents placed a great deal of importance and value on discipline, working, and climbing the ladder. Years go by, and life becomes increasingly busy, especially for parents and families. As the days go by the to-do lists only grows and other duties seem to take priority over quality family time. Oftentimes parents are misled because we do spend a large amount of time with our children; it's just not quality time. Quality time is giving your child your undivided focus and participating in activities they enjoy. It can be especially complicated for a man to choose between putting food on the table and being physically present for life's many events. On the contrary, a mother is intrinsically nurturing and inherently encouraging. Whether it's by nature or nurture, mothers typically give most of their free time to their children. And as most mothers would, Sarah had taken Dontre' to most if not all of his doctor's appointments up to this point. Living in a hospital for days at a time can be extremely

EVEN THE DARKEST NIGHT WILL END

taxing, even for the strongest of individuals. I cannot begin to count the days and nights Sarah voluntarily stayed away from the comfort of our home to provide comfort and solace for Dontre'. Needless to say, that alone is powerful. It takes a lot of strength to be a mother...a strong, assertive, yet delicate flower that, of course, is everyone's favorite. As the Creator has fashioned a mother, she is a very powerful force for her children. She is their supporter, always on their side, and willing to battle for them against all adversity. And Sarah, my beautiful wife, during these perilous and fragile moments, had blossomed into that kind of gorgeous flower.

Sacrifice is not a concept that most people genuinely enjoy unless we're on the receiving end. Although we hear the word tossed around more in modern times, most people do everything they can to avoid having to make sacrifices. It may sound ironic but we will make sacrifices in one area just to avoid having to make sacrifices in another area! This shows us that humans typically value one area of their lives more than other areas, and we would rather die than release even the smallest portion of what we love most. Most of us like to view ourselves as selfless givers but in all honesty, the very idea that we must sacrifice in a relationship enrages us. Sacrifice can look very different given the dynamics of that relationship, especially when it comes to a parent/child relationship. From a Biblical standpoint, sacrifice means to freely surrender your wants, needs, and wishes for the benefit and well-being of those you value. In retrospect, I realize that no one is actually self-made. No matter how successful, no matter how many trials a person had to overcome, someone else sacrificed for you to be here. No human in all of history can actually claim to have built themselves and their lives all on their own. In a society that encourages entrepreneurship, everyone wants to be their boss, but even the entrepreneur depends on someone. Virtually all business leaders rely on support from the government. And if you think about it, almost all of those individuals were educated at public schools or universities,

SEYMOND PERRY, SR.

or their companies rely heavily on public roads and airports, or they protected their innovative ideas through copyright and intellectual property laws. However, you look at it, no one is self-made. Parents give up a lot of things to raise happy and healthy kids. This is something children usually don't realize until they are much older and have children of their own. Raising children is a costly undertaking, not just financially, but socially, emotionally, and spiritually as well. As an adult, I can see the many sacrifices my parents made out of love for my siblings and me. But like most children, we don't actually appreciate our parents in totality until they are no longer available. Try as we might, the whole notion of sacrifice, great or small, seems so foreign to this new-aged generation.

What do today's dads most desire to learn about how to raise their children? In my opinion, the top three areas of concern for any father are understanding child development, how to cooperate with mom to raise their child, and how to discipline their child. With the world wide web at our fingertips, there is no shortage of advice or recommendations. Although fathers can oftentimes be characterized as second best when it comes to parenting, there is no substitute for a lovingly assertive dad. Although a mother's love is meaningful and unique, having an involved father figure plays an equally significant role in the healthy growth of a child. Long before the advent of the internet, there has been an underlying assumption that a father is personally involved in the training and discipline of his children. Moses ties a man's love for God with his responsibility to instill that same love in his children. *These words, which I am commanding you today, shall be [written] on your heart and mind. 7 You shall teach them diligently to your children [impressing God's precepts on their minds and penetrating their hearts with His truths] and shall speak of them when you sit in your house and when you walk on the road and when you lie down and when you get up* (Deuteronomy 6:6 - 7 AMP). A God-fearing man cannot escape the hands-on nature of biblical fatherhood in the Scriptures;

EVEN THE DARKEST NIGHT WILL END

the calling of a man is to be personally involved in all phases of his children's physical and spiritual development. But how, how do we make these difficult and seemingly impossible decisions? How can I be with all three children, ensure their physical well-being and safety, and simultaneously spur their spiritual development? While one child is fighting to live, the other two children are fighting to merely have a normal life. As any man does, we do what we believe is right at the moment and live with the consequences.

Children are much different from adults in their healthcare needs. Especially in a crisis, especially battling cancer, children require physicians that focus on their unique needs, involve their parent's opinions from start to finish, and provide spaces that are designed to be kid-sized and child friendly. Arkansas Children's Hospital did a fantastic job of forming the most suitable team for our present situation. This team was not hindered by race, culture, sex, or even age; this group was certainly the best of the best. Because of their thoroughness, we were able to wholeheartedly count on their medical expertise. Because of their proficiency and effectiveness, we were able to trust their conclusions and recommendations to the fullest. Despite their high quality of care, Dontre's health steadily continued to deteriorate. Currently, he has a chest tube inserted into his right lung to empty the cancerous fluid that constantly fills his lungs. Because so much fluid is being pulled off, doctors are pumping a specialized mixture of fluids back into his body around the clock. Frankly, they're having trouble keeping up with this constant discharge. One day he's low on this mineral, then he's too high on another substance. This has become a song and dance of sorts, and we're having trouble staying in step. And to be fully transparent, it can be tough keeping your convictions intact when you see the lifeblood of your child repeatedly vacating their body. It was one thing for Sarah to give me updated progress reports over the phone, it was something altogether different and heartbreaking to be an eyewitness to these ordeals. Before this

SEYMOND PERRY, SR.

moment, it was much easier to hear because we would pray and he would always return home. The symptoms would subside and Dontre' would be discharged. But before my very eyes lay my son who is battling fatigue, struggling physically to execute simple tasks that he previously enjoyed doing with ease. Also, it pains me to watch this vibrant child suddenly shift emotionally and only want to sleep because he was so consumed with exhaustion. In light of the situation, I desperately fought off feelings of fear, grief, sadness, anger, frustration, guilt, and anxiety. I fought these feelings so frantically because I feared the alternative. If I embrace these feelings, what does that say about me? What will that mean for my son? I'm pretty sure these feelings are normal but I don't consider myself to be normal; I'm super, extraordinary, superior, and most resilient. I tell myself over and over again, "I can deal with this! I can handle this! This too shall pass! My son shall live and not die, and declare the works of the Lord!"

Considering his digressing state, on April 21, 2021, his medical team met with Sarah, our Pastor, and myself. This meeting was to announce that we had essentially run out of options. This meeting was to inform us that, medically, there is nothing left that they could do. When your loved one has been fighting cancer and you have tried everything medically possible without success, it can be hard to know when enough is enough. You're too close to the situation and you're blinded, or fueled, by the love in your heart. You may realize logically that there's nothing else that can be done, but when has love ever been logical? Sometimes even with the best care, sometimes even with the best staff, and sometimes even with the best facility, cancer continues to spread. It's hard to accept but professionals tell you anyway, "maybe the best option for Dontre' at this point is to stop treatment. Instead, we should focus on palliative care to keep him comfortable and out of pain." But my love, my faith, and my rage will not allow me to receive this advice. Without hesitation, I brush it aside and assured them that the Anointed One would heal Dontre'. I strongly suggest that there must be something else that can be done. We have not come all this way; we have not traversed the highs and lows of despair just to give up now. Although the doctors are somewhat reluctant, they tell us of one last procedure but it would be a "hail mary". But the reality, the truth of the matter is, even this procedure is a long shot. We agree that the procedure should at least be attempted. Who knows, maybe this will be the avenue in which the Lord chooses to display His healing power. As a group, as a team, and as a family, we stand firm, fearless, and unwavering in our faith, expectancy, and confidence in our God. Our confession remains that our son is totally and completely healed from the grips of cancer. It was in that instant I had a "moment of clarity". A "moment of clarity" for alcoholics is when they come to terms with their addiction. It's the moment they realize that their drinking habits are negatively affecting every aspect of their lives. The world seemingly stood still and then, as if we were in a movie, everything around me went into slow motion. Then the voice of the Almighty was so pronounced and clear, like the voice from Mount Sanai, or the voice from the burning bush, or the voice heard on the Damascus road. The instructions were this: *"Leave everyone and everything and remain with Dontre' until he leaves the hospital."* This means I must leave my job, a challenging decision for a man that prides himself on providing. This means I must leave what I have prayed, worked, and sacrificed so hard for. This means I must leave one of the things that make me feel like a man. But, is this not the truest calling of a man, a husband, a father? There is no greater love that one can express than to give up your life, your talent, and your resource so others can live. Because Sarah has been carrying the largest weight of doctor visits and hospital stays, the Lord has chosen the perfect timing. Because mentally, physically, and emotionally she is completely exhausted. She has contributed her part and I am so very grateful. Later that evening, our pastor calls me to check on the family and our overall stability. Of the many topics we discuss, he believes the Lord wants me to stay with my son and teach

SEYMOND PERRY, SR.

Him how to walk, operate, and live by faith. And that's just what I'm going to do, teach my son until he receives his healing and leaves this hospital.

I could never express the totality and complexities of my love and admiration for Dontre. It would take all the books throughout all of mankind's history. And even then, I don't believe the message would be fully conveyed as to just what he means to me. I love all of my children no matter what; I love them without any conditions. This does not mean I promote immoral behavior, rather my passion forces me to correct and advise against all wrongdoing. I love Dontre' not only for what he is, my son, I love him because of what he compels me to become also. A better man, a more faithful husband, more kind to humanity, a better follower of Christ. Edward Bulwer said that "Love sacrifices all things to bless the thing it loves." My late father-in-law often preached that love is always sacrificial, beneficial, and unconditional. That's another lesson that I've learned through the gift of fatherhood, sacrifice. My ability to sacrifice for those I love has grown leaps and bounds. Less and less of me, more and more of the Bread of Life. I've slowly transformed into a person who is less stingy, less greedy, and more favorable toward the needs of others. The Bible goes to great lengths to compare and contrast earthly situations to spiritual realities. These stories are oftentimes referred to as parables. One common comparison is our earthly fathers to our heavenly Father. The Bishop of Souls, our loving heavenly Father, longs to communicate with us through prayer. Unlike many of our misguided and distracted parents, He always listens to us when we talk to Him. We often make the mistake of only developing a serious prayer life during times of difficulty and stress. Daily prayer can bless you, your family, and the entire world. Prayer is also a wonderful way to invite more peace into your life, help you discover your God-given purpose, and warn you of unforeseen misfortune shortly. If the Father never had my attention before, He certainly had it now. I was all ears and willing to obey His every command.

Fasting and prayer can restore and even strengthen one's intimacy with God. Many devout Christians find that fasting helps them rekindle their hunger and thirst for the King of Kings again. For someone who has struggled with pride and arrogance their entire life, fasting is also a way to humble yourself before the Lord our God. Watchman Nee says that "Sometimes it requires much prayer, fasting, and waiting upon God. For us to know the Master's will, we must lay down our own ideas and deny the activity of the flesh." Although I am a huge advocate of fasting, it was not required for me to know the will of God in this particular situation. I immediately knew that the Lord wanted me to stay with my son and be with him through the remainder of this process. I thank God daily for the church family that I am a part of and the pastor He has given us. Once our church family heard of the most recent developments, they immediately began to fast and pray on our son's behalf. With impossible odds on one hand and grave uncertainty on the other, the Perrys continue to press on. We muster every bit of spiritual and physical strength that we have and do what must be done. Even though this situation appears to be hopeless, I am extremely encouraged that I can hear the voice of the High Priest so clearly. I am reassured that even if I am thrown into the fire, He is still with me. I am encouraged that in the midst of this bleak and dismal situation, He is with me. I am encouraged that even the darkest night will end and the sun will rise.

"Life is not a matter of holding good cards, but of playing a poor hand well." — Robert Louis Stevenson

Chapter 6
We're Going to Make It

I would have despaired had I not believed that I would see the goodness of the Lord in the land of the living. 14 Wait for and confidently expect the Lord; Be strong and let your heart take courage; Yes, wait for and confidently expect the Lord (Psalm 27:13-14 AMP).

After living with a loved one with a terminal illness, you learn quite a few things. You begin to understand that the world is filled with two categories of people: those who live in constant despair and those who live on purpose for a great purpose. Those who make their daily decisions with a greater purpose in mind have limitless hope. This hope is grounded in the truth that the Lord takes pleasure in making impossible situations possible. He does all of this to display His wonderful love for us. I would have never dreamed or even imagined that I would be in this unthinkable position. Our oldest son, who is now fourteen, is in a life-or-death battle with cancer; I am doing everything I know to keep my wife, kids, marriage.....life together. It can be challenging to hear terrible news; it can be even more daunting to accept this new information as reality. No one is immune from bad news, disappointment, or calamity in life. I'm sure anyone that's experienced what we are dealing with would agree, it's dark here; it's dark and almost hopeless everywhere I look. The constant battles with depression and anxiety are slowly taking their toll on my wife. I fear displaying any sort of vulnerability or weakness; I'm afraid any perceived weakness will cause the entire family to crumble. Because of this perceived fact, the constant battles to remain motivated and encouraged have become daunting, to say the least. Our mere existence

SEYMOND PERRY, SR.

has grown into an overwhelming and completely exhausting experience. The people who are close to you, those that love you, try to say all the right words. When someone you know is going through a trying situation, individuals are often not sure what to say. Sometimes we ramble, or worse, we say nothing and avoid the person altogether because of the pronounced awkwardness. But that doesn't help at all, it adds fuel to the fire. Their absence during this complex season leaves everyone dragging around a ton of guilt because now you've isolated someone you say you love. People even make attempts to be honest and uplifting as best they can, which is completely understandable. So, the awkward words and phrases, the distant and cold shoulders all add to the grievous burden you're already handling. The actions, or lack thereof, of your close friends, only make matters worse. And again, you come to this conclusion, it's so very dark in this place, during this season of life. It's typically believed that the darkest period of the night is just before sunrise. I'm not entirely sure this is scientifically accurate, nonetheless, the noteworthy sentiment is plainly understood. Recent events and circumstances may be complex and almost intolerable, but an expected and joyful ending is soon to arrive (Psalm 30:5). Although today appears so very dim, our confidence is in the finished work of the Creator and that confidence provides us with hope for a better tomorrow.

Some people are gifted to dance; some people are gifted to swim. Some people are blessed to be great teachers, while others are gifted with iron-clad will and determination; others are gifted to lead during times of crisis and catastrophe. Those close to me would highly disagree but I've never been naturally gifted at many things. Most of the skills and abilities that I possess were worked for and earned. Reading book after book, through trial and error, through painstaking perseverance I've grown my abilities to what they are today. Although I could have never foreseen my family in this situation, the specific set of skills that I have honed over the years, and the unwavering fortitude that

EVEN THE DARKEST NIGHT WILL END

I have developed over the years, make me the right person for the job. Even during times of despair, while others shudder at having a predictable schedule, people like me continue to have a solid daily routine. Being organized and disciplined are just a few of the skills that I take great pride in carrying. During times of great stress, maintaining structure and routine are one of the few things that assisted me in feeling organized and somewhat in control. Throughout this entire ordeal, I never wanted the lives of the children to be drastically upset or turned upside down. Probably impossible, but it was certainly worth a try. Therefore, to keep some sense of normalcy, we still faithfully attend praise team practices each Wednesday evening and church services each Sunday morning. Because we're in the Praise Team, may be out of routine and religion, maybe we continued with such great devotion out of a great sense of duty and responsibility to those around us. But more than any other reason, I'm not sure how we will survive if we are not refueled and reenergized each week by the Holy Spirit and the fellowship of the saints. Surely there is great motivation and encouragement from just being in the presence of individuals who have a much different perspective of life than you presently possess. Although miles apart, Sarah and I communicate regularly, usually through text (primarily because our sleep schedules are so very different now). When I'm awake, she's fast asleep and when I'm asleep she's usually wide awake. Although it can be quite challenging, we do our best to keep a light and joyful heart. Sending each other funny memes regularly, we continue to joke and play as best we can under the present circumstances—all the while suppressing the reality that we are in an especially heavy and dreadful position. Life does offer moments of reprieve where we can genuinely rejoice and be happy, even if the moments are fleeting. Sarai finally begins attending Head Start, which provides Sarah with some level of peace and relaxation during the day. I remember Sarah sending me plenty of pictures and videos of her walking into the school with her little pink backpack. The backpack

SEYMOND PERRY, SR.

was almost bigger than she was, which we thought was outright hilarious. Of course, Dontre and I take time to look at each picture and video and he is such a proud big brother. Amazingly, he is not so concerned about himself and wants to be updated later that evening on her first day of school. And just as quickly as the excitement came, it scurried away from us. Reality slaps us in the face as we remember Dontre has a procedure on the same day, April 22, 2021. This was the "hail mary" procedure; the procedure that was a last-ditch effort to slow the bleeding and possibly save my son's life. The procedure was scheduled to be approximately 4 - 6 hours, which is a long time to sit and wait. Of course, we are always praying, but in these moments you seem to find a way to pray harder, longer, and stronger than in times past. You find a way, who am I kidding? The Power of the Highest helps you to pray more earnestly than ever before. Because the procedure is so long, or I have the attention span of a squirrel, I take the liberty of leaving the hospital to take care of some personal matters. I take this time to retrieve some faith-building artifacts for his room. Just from mere sight, these objects are intended to boost our faith. Red ribbon to place over the door (Passover), a large picture of Dontre with his siblings (a point of focus to see himself healthy and whole), the Lord's Supper (to fulfill the promise of Scripture), and Anointing Oil (in obedience to God's Word). Upon my return to the hospital, I was notified that the surgery went well and that Dontre' was resting well. I then begin the dutiful process of "decorating" his hospital room, anointing him and his room with oil, and attempting to find rest for the evening.

If there's one thing most people could use more of it's the ability to focus. To harness all of your will, emotions, intellect, and spirit towards one singular object. Telling yourself to remain focused seems pointless because no matter how hard you try, your attention seems to be drawn elsewhere. But as the days go by, as the weeks progress, every ounce of my focus and complete attention is only on Dontre' and

EVEN THE DARKEST NIGHT WILL END

his complete recovery. I quickly lose track of job security and honestly don't care. If the Root of David can heal our son, certainly He can secure my employment or provide a new place of employment. I plainly remember telling Sarah that I can find another job but I cannot find another son, at least not another Seymond Dontre' Perry, Jr. From the time I wake up until I finally close my eyes at night, every thought and action is geared towards the recovery and wellbeing of my son. Nonetheless, the Bible explains to us that there is another level of battle, of resistance, of striving (Hebrews 12:4). Certainly, there is a transformation in our way of thinking from racing to fighting. And even in this battle, we have yet to reach the point of death, dying in faith, dying because of faith, dying so that others might gloriously live. So, we press on with heaviness of heart and with a greater resolve to believe; we press on. We continue as we have countless times before. April 25 was a typical Sunday, at least a typical "hospital" Sunday. As a part of my routine, I would typically rise early on Sundays. Partly because I despise being late for anything and to accomplish everything that must be done before I attend church also. After getting dressed, I would take about 45 minutes and recite my Confession of Faith and pray. After that, I would pray with Dontre'. We would hug and kiss (which is a huge miracle for a teenager). Then I would race down the highway on the 45-minute trip back home to attend church. Just as varied as the types of church one can attend, people have a variety of reasons why they attend church consistently. Some will attend so their children have a moral foundation, while others do it to be part of a faith community. Some show up to meet new people and socialize, while some do attend to become closer to God. While all of these reasons are noteworthy, I've made it a practice to be there regularly so my family and I can receive invaluable spiritual nourishment that will keep us focused, energized, and motivated in life. Maybe I'm battle-worn or maybe I'm just anxious, but for some reason, I'm extremely anxious to return to Dontre's side. Feeling hopeless, constantly worrying, and

SEYMOND PERRY, SR.

feeling on edge can consume any individual in this kind of situation. And if left unchecked, these emotions can worsen your ability to deal with other situations well and may even damage your mental health. Attempting to be a good wife, Sarah does her best to take care of children and husband alike, as best she can under the present circumstances. Knowing from first-hand experience what I'm experiencing, Sarah encourages me to take a nap at home before returning to the hospital. And as much as I long to rest at home, I cannot calm my heart or mind enough to find rest. Some may not think of it as anxiety but the loss of control, and all humans at their core, desire control. In this type of situation, you feel continual waves of worry over your loved one. These feelings can be triggered by several things, most of which are created by a series of negative thoughts. Primarily, constantly thinking or talking about your loved one in the hospital. This pressure can reveal itself in multiple ways from racing thoughts, shortness of breath, chest pain, headaches, or even heart palpitations. In this instance, for me, stress is revealing itself as sleeplessness. And since I can't seem to find slumber, I reluctantly head back to the hospital, knowing this is the only course of action that will provide any level of comfort.

After being in this situation for what seems to be forever, some days you can wonder if you are truly seeing any improvements. Are the successes and victories so small now that it's hard to even notice them? Are we even making any headway or are we at a standstill? And we dare not think, could this circumstance honestly be getting worse? We reside in a critical stage in the process. We thank the Savior daily for even the smallest, seemingly insignificant successes. If I take my emotions out of the equation, Dontre's health does appear to be getting better day by day, no matter how incremental and we are super excited about the direction of the progress. The "hail mary" procedure is working; to our amazement, it is working! Slowly but it's working. Daily the nurses relay to us that Dontre is receiving smaller amounts of blood products. This is the news we have been praying for because this means he is losing less blood. This is an unmistakable answer to our prayers; of course, this motivates and encourages us beyond belief. As the days go by, he is looking, behaving, and functioning much better and the doctors are astounded by the miraculous progress he is making. Because his health is improving so is his disposition and our father/son bonding and conversations can resume as usual. Before his diagnosis, Dontre' had just learned about little girls and had taken a liking to them. And any little boy that's interested in girls, he will do just about whatever it takes to peak and keep their interest. One such thing he took pride in was his hair. After years of fussing and chastising him to keep his hair clean and manicured, he now takes great pleasure in the growth and maintenance he has attained. Throughout the first round of chemotherapy and radiation, he never lost any hair. This time around, Dontre' is being given a much stronger dosage of chemo. He was still a little weak, and try as he might, he was unable to personally brush his hair. So, after twisting his arm, he relented and allowed me to brush his hair. I noticed that there was more hair in the brush than usual but once again, I did not want to believe that his hair was falling out. The next day, after our devotional time, I asked if he wanted me to brush his hair again and of course, the answer was yes. And today, May 1, I confirmed that his hair was falling out. It's normal for people to feel upset about losing their hair. And understandably, I was a little upset and nervous to tell him about his hair loss knowing how he felt about it. It's not life or death but you never know how the smallest of negative news can affect a person who's already under duress. But when I presented the situation to him, and that it would be best if I just shaved his head, surprisingly he was rather excited to have his head shaved. There was such joy and pride in his voice as he explained that with a shaved head, he would be bald like his father. To know that a son is not concerned about looks, stares, or even ridicule. To know that his heart desired to be like his father. This is the longing aspiration of

SEYMOND PERRY, SR.

every father, that their child imitates them. This is even the heart of our heavenly Father. So, with warmth and joy in my heart, I shaved his head as I've shaved my own so many times before. When the job was done, we posed for a selfie to send to all who were praying for us. I wanted to keep them posted on our progress and that we were still holding strong. These are the moments that I could never imagine trading for anything. There's an astonishing saying that "behind every young boy who believes in himself is a father who believed in him first." This sentiment is a great description of the special bond between Dontre' and me. From the time he was small, he looked up to me, upholding me as a real-life superhero. And in return, I have vowed to be devoted to the role of shaping that little boy into a respectful, kind, and strong man. Astonishingly, out of all of my teaching and mentoring, of my lecturing and correction, some of the best moments we spent together were in total silence laying in a hospital bed. Undoubtedly, some of the best times in a son's life are those spent quietly with his father, learning strength in silence.

Many would characterize the effort of Sarah and myself as heroic and very sacrificial. Mia Hamm says that "It doesn't sacrifice if you love what you're doing." Do I love spending countless nights at the hospital? Do I love praying night and day until I feel as if my life is being drained from my body? Do I love fighting the never-ending thoughts of depression and surrender? Do I love seeing my son in this condition? Of course, the answer to all of these questions is a resounding no. I don't necessarily love what I'm doing, but I do love who I'm doing it for; I do love the recipient of my love, Dontre'. Sacrifice can be seen as a voluntary giving up of immediate self-interests to foster the benefits of others. This sacrificial benevolence is most often seen in family relationships, especially parent/child relationships. Jim Rohn, was an American entrepreneur, author, and motivational speaker. This astounding public speaking had such a delightfully warm personality. He is quoted as saying: "If you are not willing to risk the

EVEN THE DARKEST NIGHT WILL END

unusual, you will have to settle for the ordinary." All of us begin life intending to make our mark on the world. But after life has slapped us around a few times, we suddenly arrive at a point where we are content to just settle. Many of us falsely believe that we are succeeding, but the truth is we fear that this is the best life has to offer. You feel stuck, and to cope with this tragedy, you settle. You settle for the ordinary; you settle for mediocrity. I cannot settle for the ordinary, at least not at this moment. I cannot and will not settle for the ordinary or the usual or the customary. I will and I must sacrifice everything, the usual and the unusual, the common and the uncommon. I must give my all, even if that means giving my own precious life. If my son is to live, if his life is within my hands (as his legal and spiritual guardian), I must sacrifice my extraordinary love for his well-being.

There are countless heartbreaking stories of individuals with similar situations like ours, battling cancer. Cancer is nothing new in modern history, nevertheless, the tragedy hits and hurts differently when it affects someone you love. The story has a different meaning when it contains your child. Along this journey, one of the main differences we were allowed to see is not all men/women have a healthy support system. Unfortunately, that is the sad reality for many people with terminally ill children. Although we're experiencing great anxiety, we always had someone we could turn to in times of weakness, even if they could not fully relate. Friends, family, and church members were a constant source of strength and support. While handling our episodes of despair, we would connect with countless men and women of all ages that were all alone. And the strongest of enraged criminals are driven insane by constant exposure to loneliness. Loneliness causes the bravest of souls to feel empty, cast aside, and unwanted. During precious moments, the Spirit of God would oftentimes lead us to encourage, pray with, and motivate these lonely travelers. It was dramatically revealed to us that our hospital stays were less about us and more about shining the light of Christ for all the world to see. Another

SEYMOND PERRY, SR.

startling difference in our situation and the many others we saw was not all men/women have faith in the Son of God. Yes, they profess to believe in God. Yes, they profess that they are believers in Jesus Christ. But their actions, their walk, their talk, and even their disposition tell a much different story. Even greater than a strong support system, we relied heavily and solely on the strength of our Savior Jesus Christ. Was it easy? under no stretch of the imagination was it easy. But by faith, faith in the love of our God, faith in the finished work of the Only Begotten Son, and by our constant faith in the Holy Spirit within us, we were able to maintain and even overcome from day to day. It is only because the Lord was on our side that we were continually able to be a light shining in the darkness. Although we are not out of the woods just yet, we can see a glimmer of hope, the light at the end of the tunnel. That never-ending light that is renewed daily constantly produces hope in our hearts that even the darkest night will end and the sun will rise.

"ONCE YOU CHOOSE HOPE, anything's possible." — Christopher Reeve

Chapter 7
Hope Against Hope

In hope against hope Abraham believed that he would become a father of many nations, as he had been promised [by God]: "So [numberless] shall your descendants be." [19] *Without becoming weak in faith he considered his own body, now as good as dead [for producing children] since he was about a hundred years old, and [he considered] the deadness of Sarah's womb.* [20] *But he did not doubt or waver in unbelief concerning the promise of God, but he grew strong and empowered by faith, giving glory to God,* [21] *being fully convinced that God had the power to do what He had promised* (Romans 4:18-21 AMP).

If you would be honest, we live in very difficult and perplexing times where many people feel dreadful and afraid to believe that things will ever get better in their lives. Many people operate in what's called caution fatigue, where they're tired of hearing about the ever-approaching dangers of the world. Their purpose in life becomes stagnant by inconsistent news reports and contradictory government officials. Living with a loved one who has been diagnosed with a terminal condition can invoke numerous emotions of sorrow, heartache, and despair. If this illness persists for an extended period, they too will begin to grow weary of the constant reports of negativity. At some point, all of us have been puzzled and fearful by how much evil and calamity we witness around us. One can easily get lost in their hardships because it takes great strength to not be completely engulfed by them; it becomes even more demanding and sometimes aggravating to remain on the right path. Ultimately, the forces of evil want to turn

SEYMOND PERRY, SR.

us away from God and disconnect us from Him. While spiritually fighting for Dontre's life, I feel constantly torn between how I feel and what I know is the right thing to do. Typically, ethical struggles are seen as an internal fight between a higher moral self and an untamed dark self. This image has been famously depicted on television as the angel and the devil on either shoulder. As the voices in your head grow louder and louder, you wonder if the struggle is even worth it. I've won the treacherous battle for positive thinking yesterday only to wage another grueling battle today. Sometimes, remaining optimistic feels so useless, but no one wants to feel hopeless. Even with the grace of our Wonderful Counselor covering our lives and the Holy Spirit dwelling within us, it can still be difficult to see all the positives that life has to offer. It becomes especially difficult when you're lost in the cloudy waters of negative situations and negative thinking. Please don't misunderstand me, everyone experiences negative thinking from time to time. But for some, especially those with low self-esteem, those fighting depression, and those who are enduring a complicated season in life, overcoming negative thinking can be a massive and daunting task. As the Perrys claw their way through a treacherous cancer diagnosis, it's understandable that we would be devastated by fear and even crippled by the mere thought of the future.

Once more, Sarah and I have been called together for another meeting with medical professionals. The doctors have determined that Dontre's life-altering condition is far beyond their ability and power to stop. The medical team calmly and gently conveys to us that the bleeding has not stopped but merely shifted. Although we notice less fluid output externally, internally, his lungs are still filling with fluid at an exponential rate. This news is not what we wanted to hear and lands in our lives like a bomb, frightening and disorienting us in a way that little else can. Pray and believe as we might, we are living through a nightmare scenario. But there's something to be said about an indomitable spirit, this kind of spirit does not comprehend the meaning of surrender, quit, or defeat. In shock, amazement, and full of tenacity, I refuse to accept that I will bury my son.

"No parent should have to bury a child ... No mother should have to bury a son. Mothers are not meant to bury sons. It is not in the natural order of things." - Stephen Adly Guirgis.

This is not what the Lord has promised us and I will accept nothing less than a completely healthy son. Interactions between patients and medical professionals can sometimes be extremely challenging, especially when delivering bad news. No one wishes to cause a difficult situation but common misunderstandings, by both groups, often result in such an occurrence. I don't know if it was crazy faith or stubborn arrogance but my response must have been on the borderline of rude because I remember Sarah kicking me underneath the table. In my mind, they just didn't understand; they just didn't know Jehovah-Shammah the way my family knew Him. And against all hope, this was the moment and the situation that would prove to them that Jesus Christ the Messiah was real. Whether my statement was rude or not, I don't want to hear anything that does not align with the Word of God. I refuse to entertain any notion that contradicts what I believe. "My son shall live and not die and declare the works of the Lord." This is my heart's cry; this is my every breath; this is my total focus and determination. I've spent my entire life reading Bible stories of people gripped by impossible situations. I've spent my entire life studying that my faith in God will turn around any negative situation. I've spent my entire life believing that I will successfully pass any test if it were ever presented. Here we are, in the throes of death and despair; here we are at the doorsteps of the impossible. The word endgame means the final stage of a game such as chess when a few pieces remain in play. That's exactly where we are now, the endgame. Few pieces are left on the board and only the magnificent power of Jehovah Rapha can help us now.

When all the signs point to defeat when every fiber of your being says that you have lost and when the enemy bombards your mind with

SEYMOND PERRY, SR.

images of disaster day and night, how do you maintain your hope in the Word of God? How? There is nothing in the physical realm that has any indication that this situation can or will get any better. Unlike many others, I am fully aware that every life is eventually touched by tragedy. No one is exempt from suffering, illnesses, loss of loved ones, or sadness and grief; this includes Jesus (Hebrews 4:15). When I think about those fleeting days and lingering months, apart from the compassion of God, I'm not quite sure how we survived. Keeping our sanity intact, conducting a semi-normal life, and holding our family together is enough pressure for any normal life. Add the threat of impending death and a normal person would have fainted, resigned, and deserted their faith in Christ. Bearing the burdensome pressure of affliction, simple chores suddenly became daunting; getting out of bed, showering, and even leaving the house required Sampson-like strength. To live with despair means to wake up every morning and lie down every night with a heaviness bearing down on your soul. No matter how many hours you've slept, this feeling brings about an inescapable exhaustion. Hope is the belief that something beneficial is going to come, the idea that what is presently seen is not the end of the story. For all people of all ages, hope produces innumerable benefits. And when hope is missing or hard to find, a person's soul becomes shattered and extremely unhealthy. Ultimately, faith becomes the fuel for the weary and downcast to believe that the sun will indeed come out tomorrow. Although I may not fully comprehend, hope is trusting that Jehovah-Shalom does have a plan for me and that those plans are extremely good. After enduring this season of darkness, as clear as crystal, now I understand why Job's wife exclaimed to her husband "Curse your God and die" (Job 2:9)! It's the finite ability of humanity; it's the limited capacity of mankind. Unlike God, we cannot see the forest because of the many trees. The problems that I face seem so insurmountable; the issues that lie before me seem so impossible. This daunting circumstance of cancer has made despair a normal way of life.

EVEN THE DARKEST NIGHT WILL END

It's understandable that many people, desperate to flee the unbearable anguish generated by affliction, turn to sex, drugs, or alcohol for comfort. Sadly, when the momentary results have worn off, the problems that they sought refuge from have only grown worse.

Among many influential and life-altering lessons, playing football taught me the importance of cultivating a tenacious spirit and maintaining a positive attitude despite bleak circumstances. It comes as no surprise that those who have experienced any level of extraordinary success in life have embraced the discipline of being tough even when it's hard. Martin Luther King, Jr. says at times "We must accept finite disappointment, but we must never lose infinite hope." So even if it means standing until there is nothing left to stand on, whatever that may be, we will keep fighting with Jehovah Gibbor leading our determined assault. Times like these help us discover no matter how much Scripture we understand, no matter how brave or capable we may be, all of us face seasons when everything seems to be working against us. Life seems to be conspiring against you. Just your mere existence has become drudgery, and you only seem to solve one problem just so another one can arise. To make matters worse, these situations seem to be totally out of your control; apparently, there's nothing you can do to eliminate these struggles. And if you're not careful, you're completely overcome with a never-ending feeling of gloom, doubt, and fear. More than just the blues, I'm teetering on the edge of depression. I'm in a constant battle with the voices in your head. Am I doing everything right? Will my marriage survive another blow? Can my son overcome this obstacle? Will the Lord do the impossible in my life? Then the voices begin to argue with each other, battling for dominance and supremacy within me. Will the voice of doubt and fear ever shut up? Probably not, after all, we are marred by sin, and pain and disbelief will always be playing somewhere in the background. I may not be completely sure about the outcome of tomorrow, but today I've made the decision not to listen to the voice of skepticism and insecurity.

SEYMOND PERRY, SR.

Although that feeling of apprehension may always be there, I've chosen to ignore it. Nothing good could ever come from listening to that voice. The consequences of following that voice are far too great. And I suppose all people experience these moments at some point in their lives. All of us are attempting to grapple with our unique dilemmas and the overwhelming feelings that accompany them. Lately, the world seems to be hurling from one crisis to another. Because of this, everyone is deeply hurting and no one wants to listen to wise counsel or sound advice. We've all experienced dramatic changes in how we conduct our lives, economic uncertainty, political turmoil, as well as a wide array of natural disasters. This does not take into account the varied individual traumas that countless people are also dealing with (loss of a loved one, declining health, unemployment, divorce, violent crime, tragic accidents). For most people, this season is only a continuation of unpredictable and unprecedented struggle and devastation.

In ancient Greek, the word paraclete means 'advocate' or 'helper'. Our Paraclete is also the Holy Ghost; He is our Intercessor, our Aide, our Comforter, and our Consoler. One Holy Ghost's primary role is to aid us when life hands us more than we can handle. He supports us by providing daily spiritual power. I'm positive that it was His wonderful energy that carried us because there is no way we mustered up this kind of faith on our own. At the moment, it can be difficult to distinguish between human strength and supernatural strength. So often, humans can be tricked into believing that their strength is more than enough; when the truth is, our ability is very limited even in daily mundane circumstances. Whether it's pride or stupidity, humans foolishly think they have what it takes to handle all of life's obstacles. On the contrary, there is something special about relying on a firm foundation; a rock to stand upon when your entire world is crumbling around you. Through many failures and mishaps, I've learned I am nothing without the kindness, authority, and insight of the Holy Spirit. Another function of the Spirit of Grace is to inspire us through the various circumstances

EVEN THE DARKEST NIGHT WILL END

of life. His presence, or lack thereof, also determines the level of success we achieve. However, many people have "fought against" or "grieved" the Holy Spirit until He was rendered ineffective in their lives. The sad part is most people aren't even aware of their horrible misstep. The Holy Spirit works in and through the most unfamiliar situations; people need to understand that things are not usually as bad as they seem. He is our helper in times of confusion and chaos; He may appear as a little child or even through a song playing on the radio. From a spectator's perspective, it must have been something to behold our faith in these critical moments; it was even more spectacular to experience. With all the reasons and odds stacked against us, we knew the Word of Yahweh Shalom to be true. We knew that come hell or high water, by faith, our son was "already" healed.

You see it in the eyes of countless people as you go about your day. You perceive its absence as people lay out their plans for tomorrow and beyond. The countless visitors we meet within these hospital walls testify to this truth. You hear it in the cries of a scared mother who has no one to talk to; you see it in the faces of workers and support staff who have no real promise or ambition beyond today. They lack passion, positive expectations, or confidence and that's incredibly painful. This seemingly small thing is an invaluable commodity for the human race; that priceless asset is hope. And when you lack hope in one area, it can become extremely taxing to any area of life. In our case, marriage is what fell by the wayside. Suddenly the mood between Sarah and I became very tense, without being able to pinpoint an exact explanation for it. Gradually, day by day, this uncertainty only increased. The challenges of adultery, addiction, and separation have always been the cause of marital stress. But now, it's the possible death of our child that's brought our marriage to a new intersection. With all that being said, restoring hope in one area of life oftentimes restores hope in another area.

SEYMOND PERRY, SR.

"Hope is being able to see that there is light despite all of the darkness." —Desmond Tutu

Yes, disappointments will occur for all of us. Try as you might, create the best plans, and solidify every contingency, the sun shines on everyone and it rains on everyone as well. The truth is, if you live long enough, you're most likely going to experience several incredibly stressful events. A loved one will die. You'll get sick. Someone will mistreat you. "I'm a good person, so how could this happen to me?" is a common question people ask when tragedy strikes. Again, bad things happen to everyone. But when faced with insurmountable obstacles, we must never lose boundless hope. Hope is what wakes us each morning; hope is what thrusts us out the front door. Hope is what brings us safely home again and hope is what encourages us to do it all over again. And though the night may be long and lonesome, hope in my Father, hope in His eternal Word, it is the hope of seeing my son healthy and whole once again that keeps us moving forward. Heavy, bruised, and downtrodden, nonetheless, hope for a brighter and better tomorrow keeps us moving forward.

Everyone has moments when they feel completely helpless. Sometimes it can get so bad that you no longer want to get out of bed, and things that once brought you joy and excitement no longer spark your interest. Every day you waddle through the motions of existence, meanwhile, you're still barely engaging in your own life. You don't even have the resilience or the interest to look for moments of joy anymore. I don't think it's a course of action that I've taken intentionally. More of a coping mechanism, more of a means of survival, I've oftentimes embraced hopelessness because misery and despair feel so much better than facing the possible pains caused by defeat and disappointment. Any emotion, no matter how drastic, feels significantly more pleasing than facing the possibility of death. But when you have hope, you desire an outcome that makes life better in some manner. But hope isn't just about making a current difficulty a little more pleasant, hope

EVEN THE DARKEST NIGHT WILL END

eventually makes our lives so much better overall. By imagining a better tomorrow, we subconsciously begin taking steps in that direction. Whether you agree or not, hope is a part of everyone's life. Everyone and I do mean everyone, hopes, and dreams for something. It's a natural part of being human; it's something the Creator placed within us. Hope helps us determine what we desire and dislike in our future. It's one of the most remarkable qualities that the Father placed within us. Even in the most dismal of situations, we can look within to see a brighter tomorrow.

It's because of the despair that we face today that we gain a deeper understanding of the pains of others. And no matter how prideful or narcissistic a person may be, life's circumstances have a way of breaking our arrogance and self-absorption. On countless occasions, I've found myself at the crossroads of pretension and humility. Staring into the face of a mess that I created, a mess that could have easily been avoided if only I had listened. It's during these times that we feel the greatest sense of loss and despair. How could I be so stupid? Why am I like this? When will I ever get my life on track? What we must understand is that hope, like faith, is a choice. And like Mary, I have made a conscious decision to choose the "better" part (Luke 10:42); I've boldly chosen to remain at the feet of Jesus. Do I understand? Not entirely. Am I frustrated? Yes, beyond belief. "If the most important part of your life is ahead of you, then, even during the worst times, one can be assured that there is more laughter ahead, more success to look forward to, more children to teach and help, more friends to touch and influence. There is proof of hope...for more." (The Noticer). So, I must remain focused on the promises of God. The Spirit of the Most-High reminds me over and over again that the Father is completely aware of what I'm enduring, and He promises strength and guidance for all who trust Him. Through this devastating experience, I've learned how to hear His voice, and more importantly how to be completely obedient to His voice. I suppose this is the most complicated aspect of hardships, being

SEYMOND PERRY, SR.

able to see beyond the moment. There were times, walking around that cold hospital, I wondered would our circumstances ever change. There were times I was unable to look beyond the crisis, beyond cancer, beyond the possibility of my son dying. There were many days and endless nights that I searched the Bible cover to cover looking for a sign or a message that everything would be alright; I badly needed a sign that things would improve and get better. Heartache, pain, and frustration can become all-consuming. One of the reasons people commit suicide is because they lose all hope for a better tomorrow. The famous proverb explains "Hope delayed makes the heart sick; longing fulfilled is a tree of life." In layman's terms, the longer a person goes without seeing their hope realized, the more likely they are to become discouraged. On the other hand, seeing your hopes realized is remarkably reassuring and uplifting. It can become easy for any of us to lose perspective. And when your child has been diagnosed with a terminal illness, when you've realized victory only to have your hopes and dreams fiercely dashed before you, what else is there to do? If all you can see is right here and right now, the hospital bed, the tubes, the tears, the weakness, and distress, you will be completely downcast. But, when there was nothing left to hope in, I paused for a moment, took a deep breath for a second, and began to hope against all hope. I began to strengthen and fortify my remaining faith in the Lord my Creator, even though there was nothing physical to hope for. In that hope, I found that no matter how horrible the news or how dreadful the situation is, in those still quiet moments I can see that even the darkest night will end and the sun will rise.

EVEN THE DARKEST NIGHT WILL END

"One day at a time, one step at a time. Do what you can, and do your best. Let God handle the rest." — Michelle Jones

Chapter 8
The Darkest Night

Weeping may endure for a night, but a shout of joy comes in the morning (Psalm 30:5 AMP).

"If you're walking down the right path and you're willing to keep walking, eventually you'll make progress." -Barack Obama.

I'm certain that we are walking down the right path, praying, fasting, confessing the Word, teaching Dontre's faith, and all the other spiritual disciplines. I am positive that all of heaven is supporting us through the perilous and monstrous storm called cancer. Throughout all of recorded history, people have always been intrigued by the power of the will to live. Like all living animals, humans have a powerful survival instinct. The will to live is a force within all of us to fight for survival when our lives are threatened by an illness such as cancer. In part, this is where we get the phrase "fight or flight." Although fascinating, this force is greater in some people than in others. Though my life is not directly in jeopardy, if my son dies, I feel a part of me will die as well. Because of this, every fiber of my being screams that what we are doing must be continued and even intensified, although some of these spiritual exercises go against all logic and reason. But no matter how illogical, we are certain these actions will ultimately lead us to victory; our practice and belief will ultimately liberate my son from the clutches of cancer. When the smoke clears and the dust settles, I have faith that we will be beautifully and perfectly crowned triumphant. I'm sure of it; I am wholeheartedly depending on this truth. Although we have experienced days of great success and many nights of extreme failure, I know that my son is going to be alright.

SEYMOND PERRY, SR.

As we have traveled, we have seen, felt, and experienced the might and power of Jehovah-Rohi, the One who is ever present in every situation of life. And like the Great Shepherd that He is, His love and compassion, stability, and attentiveness have been with us through the entire process. Despite all these facts, we are yet living from day to day within a brutal nightmare. Over the weeks and months, we have made so much progress towards health and healing; still, we are paying another visit to ICU with the prognosis extremely unfavorable. As we attempt to hold on to our trust in the Highest, things don't look promising at all. I couldn't tell you exactly when circumstances shifted, but at some point during the evening, Dontre's vitals took a drastic turn for the worse. And with the drastic shift, darkness falls. It's dark outside and doubtlessly it is dark within these four walls. Greater still, it's now dark within my heart, mind, and soul. We are all alone, my Dontre' and me; alone to face the death angel that can be heard, felt, and even seen.

Experiencing darkness, especially within your soul, is a life-altering experience that many will go through at some point in their lives. Sometimes covert, other times overt, beneath the surface there is a transformation of self-taking place. This darkness of the soul can be compared to the dark and ferocious winters of Scandinavia. The harsh winters of Scandinavia can be cruel and bleak to anyone, especially outsiders. Just imagine, snow and ice as far as the eye can see, then more snow storms, accompanied by complete darkness; did I mention there's more snow? Even for the natives, from October to March things are pretty dismal. While Dontre' is the one being attacked, for this outsider, things are extremely dark. A "night" is essentially when a person loses their connection to everything they once held as valuable, to everything they once believed was true. Living through a prolonged bout with a sick loved one can often conjure up feelings that you're losing your faith. This loss of faith is not only towards; this loss is towards science, loved ones, and even myself. In other words, a "night" is a prolonged disconnection from the Everlasting God. This prolonged

EVEN THE DARKEST NIGHT WILL END

disconnect is what caused Christ to question the presence of the Father and why He felt so alone. For lack of better words, it's a spiritual crisis; it's an intense, dark period of questioning what is real, who is real, and why you even exist. These dark periods are usually brought on by something traumatic that happens in our lives, but not always. It's as if someone pulled the rug from under your feet and you aren't able to catch your balance again. You're blindfolded in a dark room, alone, and you just can't seem to find a way out.

Have you ever had someone tell you that a loved one is going to die? Sure, most of us have at some point in our lives. I believe in some respect; we all know this to be true. For it is appointed in the life of all mankind, good or evil, to leave this world. It was Charles Franklin who said, "No one gets out of this life alive." In comparison, has anyone ever told you that your child was going to die? This too is a huge possibility. Given the world that we live in, I'm sure that many of us have had to face this very real possibility. And at this moment, that is what I am faced with; every couple of hours a nurse visits us to check Dontre's vitals. There's a creepy and almost ominous seriousness within the room. "Is there anyone in your family on the way? Is his mother en route to the hospital? Do you need us to call anyone for you?" These were the questions being asked throughout the progression of this night. But even in the face of insurmountable odds, even with my son gasping for air, I refuse to let go. My love for you and God's passion for us will see us through. "I made a promise to you and I will be a man of my word; you will walk out of this hospital! You will live and not die! You will live to declare the mighty works of the God of Covenant!" This is where we find ourselves; this is the darkness that drives many strong men to insanity.

"Even a happy life cannot be without a measure of darkness, and the word happy would lose its meaning if it were not balanced by sadness."
— Carl Jung

SEYMOND PERRY, SR.

It's so very easy to believe when things look good and when all is well while standing at the pinnacle of life. The true test of faith is whether you can speak life amid impending death. Can you trust the Spirit of Knowledge when you cannot feel His presence? Can you stand strong at the helm of a sinking ship even as the flood waters continually rise? What makes this situation so much different than the others is everything around us appears to be dead. From the actions of the doctors and nurses to the looks of sadness and remorse on their faces, from the heavy and labored breathing of my son to the overwhelming heaviness in my heart. Everything around me shouts death, but everything within me says life and life much more. In any event, if it means I pour out my life as a drink offering if it means I give my last that my son might live, if it means I am consumed with eternal insanity so that he sees a bright future, I will do it. I will commit to this "foolish" course of action a thousand times over if it means my son has the opportunity to live beyond his childhood. So, against all hope, against all reasoning, against all logic, I press toward the prize. I press on through the darkest of nights; I press on with the Lord as my strength and Dontre' as my prize. I continue to pray like never before. Pray in English, pray in the Spirit, pray in tongues, pray the Holy Scriptures. I call on the name that is above every name, that is the name of Jesus Christ. I pray to the Father of lights Who hears the cries of His people and answers their prayers by fire. I innately call upon all the lessons of faith as guidance, lessons that I've studied, written, and learned long ago. I confess the Word of God over my son; I confess the Word of the King to the angels; I confess the Word of God to Satan. I recite the Word of God until there is nothing left within me to confess. I hold the limp and lifeless hand of my son, IVs, and monitors constantly beeping and buzzing. Their pesky sound is the only noise in the room that rings of life and stability. I hold his hand and speak directly to his spirit; although physically unconscious, I boldly encourage him that we will walk out of this hospital together!

EVEN THE DARKEST NIGHT WILL END

The great Chinese church pioneer Watchman Nee wrote "the Lord purposely places us in adverse circumstances to remind us that without His life we cannot stand. The power of His life is made manifest through outside pressure". The Apostle Paul says that the Lord's strength is made perfect in his weakness. Because of this, every overwhelming or pain-stricken moment of a person's life is an opportunity for the Holy Spirit to display His wonderful ability. Of course, this is not how we typically view life, at least not naturally. Our society holds individuals to an incredibly high standard of near perfection. This causes us to throw our weaknesses aside and hide our failures and shortcomings. Tragically, we put on a facade of strength that we are too feeble to keep up. When we pretend to have it all together, we've literally abandoned our truest selves. From personal experience, we do this in an attempt to control what others think about us; this facade is a foolhardy coping mechanism. So we cover, manipulate, and camouflage ourselves to gain approval from others, or to avoid their disapproval. And when it's all over, you've betrayed the most valuable person you know, yourself. While pondering these thoughts the revelation occurs to me, what I have is not enough. This substance, this life, the will to live buried deep within me, although assertive and strong, is not sufficient. It is not enough to see me safely through this treacherous night. My prayers begin to quickly shift from Dontre and his well-being, and I begin praying for my frailties and weaknesses. On the heels of this new revelation, if there is not an immediate transfer of supernatural power to me at this very moment, I will not survive. And if I don't survive, I fear that my son will not prevail either. Everything I believed before this moment seemed so simplistic and even juvenile. It felt all too easy to believe in the promises of God. "If God said it, I believe it and that settles it." But here, within these moments of rejection and solitude, within the darkness, I find my faith slowly slipping away. Where do you go when you can't see or hear or even feel the presence of the Almighty? Who do you turn to

SEYMOND PERRY, SR.

when you question every decision you've made up to this point? When emotions run high and trust runs low, exactly how do you regain a firm grip on reality?

Another quote from Watchman Nee says: "To pray through and to pray with strength is not a vain expectation. Ease and comfort will not get us into this prayer life, and neither will we ever drift into this prayer life. We must learn a little, break a little, and fight a little to obtain such prayer." And maybe, just maybe, this is what the Lord intends for me to learn....how to effectually and fervently pray. Within this call to prayer, I've lost all track of time and reality. The only thing that snaps me back to reality is the scheduled visits from the medical staff. Still, the nurses persist, like clockwork, they question if Dontre's mother would be joining me tonight. Proudly, I insisted that she would not be needed tonight because my son would live to see her tomorrow. And as the nurses quietly exit the room, I return to a posture of humility and sobriety before a Sovereign God. In retrospect, I've never prayed this deeply or this forcefully in my life. During times of peace and security, we are delusional to believe we are praying with all our minds, body, and spirit. Times of crisis cause us to go further, dig deeper, and stretch further than ever before. It's not until your back is against the wall that we really answer the call to launch out into the deep (Luke 5:4). You've sought the Lord and you still see no change, no evidence, no confirmation, no manifestation. After all of my searching, there is still no positive witness within my spirit. So, as any loving father would do, we oppose the forces of darkness once more; we remain steadfast in our convictions and pray without ceasing. And when there is nothing left, when the tank has run empty of spiritual fuel, when we are empty and have no more life or stamina within ourselves, we know that we must carry on. We only afford ourselves the smallest of breaks. These few moments of escape are merely designed to refresh and re-energize us spiritually, nothing more. We scurry to the nearest restroom to seek the Lord for continued determination and fortitude in the face of death

EVEN THE DARKEST NIGHT WILL END

itself...''Lord, I am so tired; I am so broken, I am so empty. I cannot survive this moment without Your intervention. Fill me again with your precious Spirit of Life. By faith, I receive You again that I might complete the assignment that is laid before me." And just like the ten lepers cleansed by Chief Corner Stone, as I walked back to Dontre's room, He would always refill me, pour into me rivers of living water, revive the dry bones, and stoke the flickering embers of faith within me. All concerns for the physical man (food, rest, basic hygiene) have been cast aside many hours ago. Heart and soul are all that remain. If this task is to be accomplished, if my son is to walk out of this hospital, success will only be achieved by the supernatural power of the Savior. During these invaluable moments, just like in Alice in Wonderland, we travel down a road that leads us further and further away from the physical realm. Not sure whether I passed or fell asleep, whether praying in the spirit or if we had finally serum to exhaustion, what I do know is when I opened my eyes the glorious sun was just peaking over the distant horizon. With a rough and shaky voice, the sweetest sound welcomed the new day. Dontre gazed at me with fondness and all sincerity: "Hey dad!" I'm immediately overcome with a host of feelings and emotions. Joy, relief, happiness, pride and so much more are felt from the mere sound of his voice. With tears in my eyes: "Hey son, we made it. Last night was a little rough but we made it." James Weldon Johnson's words are more visibly seen, felt, and grasped: "Facing the rising sun of our new day begun let us march on till victory is won." With the rising of the sun, I've come to a renewed sense of peace and hope. Being able to see Dontre' alive, active, and alert has almost entirely restored any faith that was lost during the night. As if he didn't just wake up, I instructed Dontre' to get some rest and that I would return to his side shortly.

This incident, this dark night, was so perilous that I cannot begin to express in words what I feel. It was more than depression, more than anxiety; the weightiness of the moments was far greater than

SEYMOND PERRY, SR.

anything I'd ever felt before. This event pierced so much deeper than any heartbreak or disappointment. Approximately 70% of adults live through at least one traumatic experience in their life. Having to stand on the watch for the life of my loved one reframed everything I thought I knew about spiritual warfare. As much sorry and discomfort as I experienced on this night, there was an inner transformation and a broadening of my spiritual ability. Although best known for his artwork, Leonardo da Vinci had this to say about love. "Love shows itself more in adversity than in prosperity; as light does, which shines most where the place is darkest." It is in this dark hour that this father's love is shining brightest. A father and his affection are so crucial to the overall well-being and stability of the home. When he is absent (mentally, spiritually, emotionally), his void devastates the mother and the children. A dad is an anchor upon which his children stand. I am that anchor; I must be stable and secure against all enemies, domestic and foreign. With the Holy Spirit as my source, I must stand strong against all opposition. When the Lord moves, as I know He will, He will see faith residing within me.

Most people would now feel a sense of relief and be at ease after this victorious chain of events, but PTSD is a very real and difficult affliction for many people. PTSD usually emerges after any type of traumatic event. Against all odds, we made it through the night but I am completely and utterly drained. On the other side of victory, all of those feelings of fear, dread, and terror are now flooding me all at once. Unknown to me at the time, I am experiencing the beginning stages of Post-Traumatic Stress Disorder. Feelings of mistrust, insecurity, and worry over time my heart and mind. I've fought so hard for Dontre' that there is now nothing left for me to defend myself. I feel no love; I feel no connection to the world around me; this includes being connected to the Father. Just like Elijah, I feel isolated and frustrated; being "stuck" here I feel powerless to change the circumstances I face. I frantically scroll through my phone looking for someone to call. After

EVEN THE DARKEST NIGHT WILL END

exposure to kryptonite, even Superman cries out for help. I look at several names and ponder what they would or could possibly do to help me at this moment. Maybe it was pride that kept me from calling my pastor, and maybe it was keeping up a macho facade that kept me from calling my wife. In the end, with trembling hands and water-filled eyes, I decided to call my best friend, Aaron. It was still early so I was not surprised he did not answer. I scroll through my contact list again looking for someone I believe will not only sympathize with me but also encourage me through this difficult moment. Maybe personal preference or maybe the Lord, but I called my Aaron's wife believing she would answer the phone and she did. At the brink of falling apart, with fear and worry in my voice, I ask to speak to him. It took her a few moments to wake him, and a few moments more for him to respond. He asks what's wrong, what did the doctors say, is everything ok? Maybe he thought Dontre' had passed during the night or that the doctors had given me another negative report. Despite the reason, no words will proceed from my lips, only heavy sobs of fear, dread, and anxiety. "I don't want my son to die. I don't want my son to die. I don't want my son to die." Within my voice, there is a desperate plea for help! Please, someone, help me save my son. I've given all I have and I don't know what else to do. He asked if I needed him there with me. And like a frantically lost child, I said yes. He assured me that he would get to me as soon as possible. It took him about an hour and a half to make it to me but just his presence was able to bring calm to my heart and mind. He wanted to visit Dontre' for himself but because of COVID restrictions, he was not allowed to come into the room. We sat on a bench outside the hospital and watched the people walk by. We briefly discussed the situation with Dontre' and how was I coping with it all. We continued to make small talk for several minutes and I'm truly grateful for his loyalty to me. Because of his friendship, for those few moments, my son was not in the hospital; I was not facing the challenge of a lifetime. I was merely sitting with my friend and having a

SEYMOND PERRY, SR.

normal conversation. We eventually left the hospital to have breakfast, which was probably best for me at the moment. We laughed, joked, and talked about the Word of God as was customary for us. It was in these moments, fleeting as they were, I grasped the truth that my son did not die last night. The doctors, the nurses, and even the devil were convinced that the story of Dontre' was finished. Once again, with weary bodies and heavy hearts, with concerns and many unanswered questions, the life of my son has been spared. When you've lived in a dark place for an extended period, it may take a close companion to help you celebrate the new beginning that each day brings; it may take a dependable friend to help remind you even the darkest night will end and the sun will rise.

EVEN THE DARKEST NIGHT WILL END

"Hope is like the sun, which, as we journey toward it, casts the shadow of our burden behind us." — Samuel Smiles

Chapter 9
To the Bitter End

This calls for the endurance of the saints, who keep God's commandments and keep faith in Jesus. *13 And I heard a voice from heaven say, "Write this: Favored are the dead who die in the Lord from now on." "Yes," says the Spirit, "so they can rest from their labors because their deeds follow them"* (Revelation 14:12 - 13 CEB).

Orson F. Whitney has the most astounding and encouraging words for parents. "You parents of the willful and the wayward! Don't give them up; don't cast them off. They are not utterly lost. The Shepherd will find his sheep. They were His before they were yours - long before He entrusted them to your care, and you cannot begin to love them as He loves them." Although profoundly accurate, this statement can be very challenging to receive; nonetheless, it's true. Whitney's argument is hard to accept because a child is one of the most critical things in a parent's life. Any emotion or feeling connected with our child only intensifies as they grow older. No pride is more incredible than watching them thrive; no despair is more heartbreaking than seeing them suffer; no pleasure is more enjoyable than sharing in their happiness. These sentiments only begin to sum up the way a parent feels about their children. Unlike any other relationship, the love a parent holds for their child can be almost indescribable. Although parental love is communicated in many different ways, at the core of each parent is a strong desire to do what is best for their child. Only when we comprehend a parent's love for their child that we start to glimpse our Advocate's love for His children. As much as I love my son, God loves him more and loves him better. The Lord loves my family with

SEYMOND PERRY, SR.

pure and selfless love. Our human frailty cannot begin to understand or display a devotion like this; His love is truly incomprehensible. Although it's foreign to us, this is the foundation of my faith and the reason for my relentless hope. May 10 was a day when my faith was stretched, questioned, and put on trial. Things are more intense than usual, dealing with a tough and demanding projection, unexpected disappointments, and a grim tomorrow. It's in these moments God's love for me can seem so very distant and almost doubtful. In these moments, how am I supposed to be living in these trying moments example of faith in these moments? How do we relinquish control of the plans we have for our child's life? Even when His plans seem contrary to our dreams and aspirations, how do we trust God's plans instead? Honestly, I don't know all the answers, but our Sovereign God has a way of grounding us, comforting us, and inspiring us to stay devoted.

Through Biblical testimony, we can see that pastors are strengthened by the confidence members have in them. This trust is usually earned or forfeited during the critical moments of their lives. One of the many duties that befall a pastor is visiting discouraged members during times of personal crises. There is such a blessing extended to family and friends from pastoral visits. When the Lamb of God physically lived on earth, He paid close attention to visiting people within the community (going house to house, healing the sick, comforting the mourners, soothing the afflicted, and speaking peace to the brokenhearted). In response to the severity of Dontre's situation, our pastor has scheduled an appointment with Dontre'. In pastoral ministry, it can often feel like the days are filled with agonizing dilemma after agonizing dilemma. A huge part of shepherding the flock of the Chief Shepherd is caring for the hurting and broken as they face the adverse obstacles of life. Like any good teacher, he knows what we've been taught and is well aware of our capabilities. He believes we are well able to see our son delivered from the cold grips of the ICU

EVEN THE DARKEST NIGHT WILL END

to the warm embrace of our family and friends back at home. I'm sure our pastor is confident in our spiritual fortitude, maturity, and ability; nonetheless, he still must fulfill them as well. Throughout this entire process, Pastor Robertson has taken great efforts to keep the lines of communication open. Whether through text, phone calls, or in person, our pastor was certain to stay abreast of the family's mental, physical, and spiritual well-being. During his individual prayers, there were many occasions when he would relay direct instructions from heaven to me. Whatever God tells us to do, He will always verify the instructions from His Word. Then, because He knows the frailty of humanity, He will confirm it to us - oftentimes through repetition. Time and again his words were only validation of what I was already hearing or doing with our son. As I expected, our pastor conducted many of the same spiritual routines and practices that we had implemented. Even though I pride myself on being a studious pupil, some lessons are only fully realized while "in the trenches". Johann Goethe left on record that "Knowing is not enough; we must apply. Willing is not enough we must do." The inventory of teaching strategies is ever-expanding as there are numerous ways for us to acquire and retain wisdom. The technique of learning by doing has been around for a long time and is surprisingly effective. Regardless, our pastor was standing in Dontre's hospital room at the moment. As a remarkable under-shepherd, he was very observant, kind, and supportive. He gave our family great praise for the strength and stamina that we had exhibited thus far. Also, he gave a significant compliment that will always stand out in my mind. "There are so many things that I see your family has done during this time, even within this hospital room that are commendable. In the past, I've had to guide families through the faith process step-by-step, but not the Perrys. This family has put everything in place to encourage and promote a great move of God." And that's exactly what we need, that's exactly what we are believing for - a miracle. More than ever before, we desperately need the supernatural intervention of God. Because

SEYMOND PERRY, SR.

humans are always in trouble, all of us have needed a miracle, need one now, or will need one in the future. The issue is that most Christians don't know how to even begin receiving a miracle from Emmanuel.

Although I consider myself to be a very tough guy, no one at any stage of life should live in constant pain, especially a child. Because he is experiencing so much discomfort, from breathing to basic bodily functions, Dontre's pain medications were extremely strong. For hospice patients struggling to breathe, which is our current condition, small amounts of well-controlled morphine can help ease respiratory distress and alter how the brain responds to pain. Also, these medications ease the stress and anxiety of laboring to catch one's breath. But with a little coaxing, we were able to get Dontre' to wake up. And with a little more coaxing, we were able to get him to a place where he was mentally alert. But when it was all said and done, he listened to the encouraging words of our pastor and received them with great joy and belief. Several scriptures were recited and expounded upon; several words of wisdom and advice were given to me as well as the family. When spoken with truth and sincerity, encouragement goes straight to the heart. I don't think most people realize the huge difference they can make in the lives of others. While encouragement is something everyone wants and needs, not everyone knows how to receive encouragement properly. As his father, I was so proud of Dontre' for how he respected the words of our pastor. A father never underestimates the abilities of their children; they're always striving and pushing their kids to higher greatness. Not only was he receptive but he also attempted to do everything that was asked of him. Sometimes it is nigh impossible to convince a proud father that their beloved offspring is incapable of doing anything. In any event, afterward, we partook in the Lord's Supper (a daily practice for Dontre and me). The word crisis simply means you've come to a crossroads. A crossroad is a place of decision. In a crisis, you must decide how you will respond. And when you and I come to that crux, that decision point

EVEN THE DARKEST NIGHT WILL END

in the crisis, we must be mindful that every crossroad reminds us of the cross of Jesus Christ and His triumph. When we keep the cross in proper perspective, we ultimately find our solution. With Christ in our hearts, with Christ in our minds, with Christ proceeding from our lips, we held hands and prayed. Although we live a life of Godly devotion, these challenging times call for the fervent prayers of God's people.

After he completed the task he came to perform, I happily escorted our pastor to his vehicle. Probably the most familiar metaphor in the Bible for the responsibility of a pastor is that of a shepherd, and the comparison is a suitable one. Everyone can picture a shepherd caring for his sheep and how that relates to caring for people. The body of Christ must always remember that pastoral care is of utmost importance to God. This calling is something He ultimately uses to impact the lives of Christ-followers forever. Seeing that I was outside, I decided to make a quick trip to the store for a few essentials Sarah and I needed. It comes as no surprise that when a loved one is sick your well-being can be significantly affected as well. Living in a hospital for days at a time, without the comforts of home, self-neglect takes place rapidly and when you're acting as a caregiver for that family member, there's also mental and emotional fatigue that wanes heavily as well. While at the store, my heart was still heavily concerned about Dontre' and whether he was resting well. So, at 2:00 PM, I texted Sarah to see if physical therapy would be continued although he was officially in hospice. There are no easy answers when a loved one has a serious illness, especially when the medical staff has run out of options to keep them alive. Sarah's response was "I just asked". And for me, no news is always good news. A few minutes later she sends me a list of personal items she needs from the store. Now a quick trip to the store has turned into an even longer trip. I suppose under the circumstances, time is really exaggerated in one direction or the other (fast or slow). Another notification from my phone, it's now 2:44 PM. Sarah has sent a picture of six doctors surrounding Dontre's bed. I'm so accustomed

SEYMOND PERRY, SR.

to seeing a swarm of doctors that the picture isn't even alarming to me. At least once each morning we have this kind of visitation. I'm very puzzled by the picture but continue shopping as quickly as possible. A few moments later, another notification from my phone. Sarah is now asking me "how much longer I would be?" Before I could type out a proper response she is calling; this is not a good sign. Have you ever heard of the 7% rule? It states that only 7% of communication is verbal and the other 93% is non-verbal and that 38% of communication is the tone of voice, but that still leaves 55% that's down to body language. This means every time you make a phone call you are only ever able to convey a maximum of 45% of your intention to the recipient down the line. But after all these years, I know this tone of voice. I know exactly what this means; I know I'm needed at the hospital as quickly as possible.

Is this it? Is this the ending of the war so bravely fought? Is this how we shall leave this hospital? As I enter the room, everything and everyone lay quiet, dormant with the stitch of death lingering near. The looks on everyone's faces say all that I need to know. He's dying and there's nothing anyone can do to save him.

"And we wept that one so lovely should have a life so brief." – William Cullen Bryant

My thoughts are moving at light speed and I'm unable to gain control of a single one of them. Although I've experienced death before, all sorts of feelings are rising to the surface. Standing there at his side, Dontre's transition is causing agony and pain that is indescribable. And the longer this departure lingers on the more intense these feelings become. Moment by moment we watch as his breathing slowly dwindles to nothing. My mind screams that this is not real; my mind yells violently that this is only a dream and I will wake up soon. My son is supposed to bury me; why am I witnessing this horrific event? In an attempt to preserve what's left, my instincts tell me to run and flee the scene of the crime. Alas, my legs are too weak and my love is too strong. No one can be an overcomer without being a prayer warrior. For one to be truly an overcomer before God he must learn to pray the prayer of authority (The Prayer Ministry of The Church: Watchman Nee - Christian Fellowship Publishers, Inc. - 1973). But at this moment, with my wife and doctors all around, there are no words I can find to adequately express what I'm feeling as the life of my son slowly and gently leave his body. Watching a loved one die is a terrible and challenging experience. While you desperately attempt to cling to the memories of them being strong and healthy, these memories become marred by this tragic ending. Try as I might conjure up some sort of faith, some sort of prayer, the faintest amount of authority, there is nothing left within me. Although my love desires to press on, my spirit says this is the end and you must help your son transition as peacefully as possible. A steady rotation of doctors and staff transition in and out of the room to pay their final respects and he struggles to take his final breaths of air.

Helpless, I glanced around the room to see if there was someone else more fitting to carry this burden, even if just for a moment, even just a minute. Is there someone that could help me, to offer some sort of relief, but there was none? Perhaps the greatest hurdle of leadership is the constant concern that leaders often must carry. This uneasiness must be heavily monitored and balanced through internal and external systems. As a husband and a father, you're a leader 24/7, whether you like it or not. When you're the leader, the final responsibility lies with you. This is both a blessing and a curse. This is the position that I've been thrust into; to understand leadership is to realize that you can't have one without the other. This is the burden of leadership. As sorrow, grief, and despair swept over her, Dontre's doctor kneeled at his bedside. She began to weep bitter tears. Maybe she felt there was more that could be done; maybe she felt like a disappointment to the family; possibly she wept solely because the life of an innocent child was slowly fading away. But in all sincerity of heart, we knew there was nothing

SEYMOND PERRY, SR.

that anyone could possibly do at this point. I examined the gorgeously brown eyes of my wife; I believed I would find the solace or the place of refuge that I'd found so many times before. Alas, she had no words to offer, no encouraging look, and there was no pep talk given to me. Every wife desires a feeling of security from her husband. Since Adam and Eve, man has provided for and protected his family. A husband must give his wife a feeling of stability; no matter what happens, she needs to know he's going to make everything okay. And at this moment with a dying child, she only gave me the look that a wife gives a husband. The look that says, "I need you to step forward, take the reins, and lead." But how can I lead, how can I with this distressing void in my soul? Have you ever had this overwhelming feeling of emptiness? Right there in the middle of your chest is where it normally occurs. You know how it got there; you are fully aware of what caused it. So empty that it's becoming difficult to breathe. Is it despair? Is it desperation? Is it a warning for the things that are to come? All I know is that I do not currently have what it takes to deal with this level of agony, this level of grief, this level of ministry. At the end of the day, we are all programmed to avoid discomfort and chase pleasure. So, when things get complicated and overwhelming, it's natural to have a deep need to just run away from it all. I quickly excuse myself to the bathroom for a moment of relief. And for a moment, it was just me and my Father. In those brief moments I inquired of the Lord, "what shall I do? Shall I pursue? Shall I speak life? What shall I do?". My son is dying, what is your will? *"Do what I've taught you to do. Speak the Word only"* (Matthew 8:8). And with those words, the room went silent, a peace that surpasses all understanding came over me, and I bravely proceeded back to my son's side. In the power of the Spirit of Wisdom, covered by the blood of Jesus, held together by the grace of Almighty God, we gracefully ushered our son into the presence of the Father. As I held his right hand as his mother held his left, the Spirit of the Living God spoke through me the infallible Word of God. Seemingly endless

EVEN THE DARKEST NIGHT WILL END

scripture after scripture began to flow from me, verse after verse, and in some moments, chapter after chapter. I continued to speak the Holy One of Israel's Words over Dontre' until he took his final breath.

Seymond Dontre' Perry, Jr. passed away from breathing complications on May 10, 2021, at 4:38 PM. C. JoyBell C. maintains that "Ends are not bad things, they just mean that something else is about to begin. And many things don't end anyway, they just begin again in a new way. Ends are not bad and many ends aren't an ending; some things are never-ending." It is from this moment, from this horrendous event, even from this painful circumstance that we now stand. Although my son did not physically survive Mediastinal Adenocarcinoma, I don't know of a braver, stronger, gentler person, and that's not just his father talking. Anyone who saw this beautiful child playing video games would say the exact thing. Anyone who watched him plays piano or guitar, or sings to our God would say the exact thing. Anyone who watched him relinquishes his last carnal ability... drawing, walking, eating, talking with such humor and grace, would say the exact same thing. That's not to say that he was perfect, none of us are perfect, not by any stretch of the imagination. But I pray that in some way, large or small, our lives have made a difference in the world. Even with my many mistakes and shortcomings, there is no mistaking my love and devotion for Dontre. Richard Paul Evans says "the depth of love is revealed in its departure." More than anything, this is the hard part, the departure; leaving behind and starting anew, the difficult part is the transition into something new and unfamiliar. Now that he is no more, at least in the way we can recognize, the feelings of admiration and affection are overwhelming. They consume our very thoughts, our hearts, our dreams, and even our words. You find yourself questioning the Great Physician, your beliefs, and everything that you've ever been taught about spiritual warfare. You question why didn't our faith, and our belief system work. Why am I here holding a cold hand while others with much less faith, much less service, and

SEYMOND PERRY, SR.

much less honor are still living and enjoying their children? Why is my love being tested while others still go unchecked? These are the depths that my love, the love I have for my son, has brought me to. And now, where I am, only God Himself can rescue me.

It can be easy to wonder why these series of abnormal events occurred in life. I believe it's human nature to have questions, fears, and even doubts. "Is there anything we could have done differently to alter the outcome that we now face?" The great evangelist, Oswald Chambers, often spoke of the Teacher's engineering circumstances. "When once the saint begins to realize that God engineers circumstances, there will be no more whine, but only a reckless abandon to Jesus." "God engineers our circumstances as He did those of His Son; all we have to do is to follow where He places us. The majority of us are busy trying to place ourselves. God alters things while we wait for Him." No, we do not blame our heavenly Father for any of these circumstances or events. He always has been and forever shall be a good Father and only delivers blessings and favor to our lives. On the contrary, we must not forget that we have a sworn enemy. This enemy to God and all those who love darkness, does not play fair and does not play according to the rules. But El Shaddai, knowing the ending from the beginning, saw this moment through all of eternity. Because of this, He has determined to strengthen us, shape us, and mold us into something better, something more powerful, and something more useful. "We are the sum of all the moments of our lives - all that is ours is in them: we cannot escape or conceal it" Thomas Wolfe expresses. Because this is true, even this heartbreaking, world-chattering event adds another layer to who I am and adds to who we are as a family. These events draw us closer to each other and closer to the loving Father. I am now able to have a new and profound appreciation for my family, for this life, and my purpose while on earth. No words can express the agony and pain my son was living with, but from the halls of

EVEN THE DARKEST NIGHT WILL END

eternity, his works and his legacy proclaim to us that even the darkest night will end and the sun will rise.

"There is no real ending. It's just the place where you stop the story."
-Frank Herbert

Closing

"Extraordinary afflictions are not always the punishment of extraordinary sins, but sometimes the trial of extraordinary graces." — Matthew Henry

Matthew Henry's Commentary on the Whole Bible. But at that moment, in the middle of the hurt and pain, while the anguish remains very real and very present, it never feels that way; it never feels like grace. You mean to tell me that it's a good thing that I, we, endured this catastrophic event. This grace, like many other blessings from the Lord, is an almost unbearable weight and burden to carry. If all of us were truthful, no one wants a life of calamity and torment; no one! There isn't one person on earth who's filled with a yearning for the various disasters of life, the ups and downs, the heartaches, and disappointments. No one ever said: "When I grow up, I want to endure the greatest sorrows and miseries of all time"! Humans don't enjoy pain; humans don't pursue affliction; humans don't rejoice in oppression. The notions and reality of hurt and suffering are very complex and multifaceted; pain contains physical as well as psychological components. Emotional pain can oftentimes feel just as strong as physical pain and at times can cause symptoms of discomfort throughout the entire body. And the stress and anxiety caused by the death of a loved one are no different. In the days, weeks, and months that followed the passing of my son, I would verbally say that I was doing alright. I'm not sure if this response was given as a brave facade; I'm not sure if this response was given in ignorance because of how a sick person properly diagnoses their illness. Regardless of my verbal response, my body, my mind, and my spirit told a completely different story. Some mornings I would wake up with flu-like symptoms and

SEYMOND PERRY, SR.

other mornings I would wake up with waves of depression showering over me. From one extreme to the next, there are just no words that can describe this new world I now lived in, a world without my beloved son.

As much as we fight against it, the human spirit is best improved upon when given regularly scheduled prescribed doses of discomfort, anguish, sorrow, and disappointment. It's like the tree that survives a terrible storm; the roots only grow deeper and stronger after each attack. It's like a muscle that only grows stronger after each bout of exercise; it's like the human spirit, that refuses to surrender, that refuses to retreat, but only grows stronger after each of life's heavy blows of disappointment and discouragement. I've taken the time to outline many of the challenges, obstacles, and detours that we faced along this journey. What I did not convey was the soon-to-follow journey of grief and the process of keeping a broken family together. If there's one thing about grief that everyone understands it's the hurt and it sucks. Sorrow is universal. Simply seeing images of someone crying over the remains of a lost loved one and you immediately feel their pain. At some point, everyone will have at least one encounter with anguish. Grief is also very personal. Like love languages, everyone experiences and conveys grief differently. It doesn't present itself tidily like a birthday present. Grief doesn't follow a given set of rules, timelines, or specific schedules. Just earlier today I was crying hysterically, but just yesterday I was furiously angry. A week ago, the despair and emptiness were so great that I was withdrawn from everyone including God. The great hope is that none of these things are unusual or even wrong. Oftentimes people try to tell others how to grieve the loss of a loved one, but honestly, there is no right or wrong way to miss someone you've loved so dearly. And I have no idea when the pain begins to subside. I couldn't tell you exactly when I could confidently lift my head again. I know that a huge focus for me was my family and not my personal well-being. My prayers now were centered around my wife and remaining children.

EVEN THE DARKEST NIGHT WILL END

And because of this, the attention to personal discomfort was somewhat negated. But like a bad toothache at midnight, when the world was quiet and the house was still, my "demons" would come out to play. Some nights I had no words but only tears, tears of sadness, tears of sorrow, tears of anger, and tears of disbelief. And though I am generally an extremely positive person, even I asked the Lord, when will the sun shine again?

The familiar saying goes "You never miss your water until your well runs dry"! We never truly know how much we love someone until we're painfully faced with the agony of their departure. Until they are gone and out of reach, beyond our physical touch, we never comprehend the height, depth, or breath of our devotion to someone. And it wasn't until Dontre' passed away, it wasn't until I could no longer hold his young hand or hear his tender voice that I realized just how much I loved him. You never recognize how far you will travel to prove your love, especially when it's your child. Although we say powerfully sophisticated phases, sometimes words just don't do it. You can preach night and day that you love them, but if actions don't align with words, no one is going to believe you. It's so easy to take the Lord's blessings for granted, our children in particular. Before you know it, the very ones you would lay down your life for feel unloved, neglected, and unappreciated. The transition of a child has a way of putting life in perspective; never again will we take for granted a single moment spent with our children.

"People you love never die. That is what Omai had said, all those years ago. And he was right. They don't die. Not completely. They live in your mind, the way they always lived inside you. You keep their light alive. If you remember them well enough, they can still guide you, like the shine of long-extinguished stars could guide ships in unfamiliar waters." — Matt Haig

How to Stop Time. This manuscript is my way of keeping my son's life, love, and legacy alive. It's a way for him to guide others as they

SEYMOND PERRY, SR.

traverse the difficult situations of life. Again, I can't tell you exactly when it happened, but it did. I don't know exactly how it happened, but it did. With the passing of each moment, each day, each month, and sometimes each year, you realize that there is more strength, more stamina, and more perseverance than you ever had before. Though bruised and battered, even battle-scarred, you are forever changed by your life experiences. You have been changed for the better; you are a completely new creature. Your life, your story is now a testimony of how our troubles, our obstacles, and even death work for our benefit. And long after the waves have calmed and the skies have cleared, when tear-stained pillows have been properly washed and put away, I am fully convinced and assured that even the darkest night will end and the sun will rise.

EVEN THE DARKEST NIGHT WILL END

"... to be a true revolutionary, you must understand love. Love, sacrifice, and death."
-Sonia Sanchez

Appendix

Confession of Faith (*6/29/2020*)

My physical body was purchased by the precious blood and awesome sacrifice of Jesus and it is no longer mine, but the Father's. Jesus Christ has borne my sicknesses and carried my pain. He was stricken, smitten with God, and afflicted for me. He was wounded for my transgressions and He was bruised for my guilt and iniquities. The chastisement needed to obtain peace and well-being for me was upon Him, and with the stripes that wounded Him, I am healed and made whole. I, along with everyone in my household, now have perfect health in our bodies. I fear the Lord and I prolong my days. I keep my heart with all diligence for out of it flows the issues of life. I have a merry heart and it does good like a medicine. My belly is satisfied by the fruit of my mouth, and with the increase of my lips, I am filled. Death and life are in the power of my tongue, therefore, I speak the life-giving words of God and I receive life and health in my body.

I will not let the Word of God depart from before my eyes, for it is life to me; for I have found it and it is health and healing to my flesh. I am justified by my words. I have the faith of Jesus Christ in me, for Jesus is in me, and He is the Author and Finisher of my faith. I speak to the mountains of sickness and disease and they obey my words and leave. I have authority and power over all disease and sickness; I command them to leave and they obey my words. I lay my hands on the sick and they recover.

My body is the temple of the Holy Spirit and all the fullness of God dwells in me. I glorify my God, Adonai, in my body and in my spirit which is His. I sow to the Spirit and reap of the Spirit life everlasting. I sow words of health and healing every day and daily reap health in my physical body.

SEYMOND PERRY, SR.

It is the will of God that I should prosper and be in perfect health even as my soul prospers.

Scripture References:

1 Corinthians 6:19-20; Isaiah 53:4-5; 1 Peter 2:24; Proverbs 4:23; Proverbs 10:27; Proverbs 17:22; Proverbs 18:20-21; Proverbs 4:21-22; Matthew 12:37; Hebrews 12:2; Mark 11:23; Matthew 10:1; Mark 16:18; 1 Corinthians 6:19-20; Ephesians 3:19; Galatians 6:8-9; 3 John 2

EVEN THE DARKEST NIGHT WILL END

Letter to Dontre's Teachers (*10/12/2020*)
Good afternoon! This is Sarah Perry, Seymond Perry Jr's mother! His father Seymond Perry is copied on this email as well!

First I want to thank each of you for working with Dontre during this challenging time! I decided to make a group email to keep all 7 of his teachers informed when he has doctor appointments that keep him from logging in to virtual class or why he hasn't logged on to either learning platform!!

I have spoken with some of you via email or on the phone but to clear up any questions, Dontre was diagnosed with adenocarcinoma back in June! He started chemotherapy and radiation back in August! He completed his radiation and chemo on the 30th of September!

He's currently being admitted at ACH due to some challenges he's having, we've been in the ER since this morning and I do not know how long he will be admitted! Thank you guys again! If you have further questions my phone number is 870-592-XXXX.

Revised Confession of Faith (4/10/21)
God's Word on Victory

A happy heart is a good medicine and a joyful mind causes healing, but a broken spirit dries up the bones (Proverbs 17:22 AMP).

Yet in all these things we are more than conquerors and gain an overwhelming victory through Him who loved us [so much that He died for us] (Romans 8:37 AMP).

Bless and affectionately praise the Lord, O my soul, and do not forget any of His benefits; 3 Who forgives all your sins, who heals all your diseases; 4 Who redeems your life from the pit, Who crowns you [lavishly] with lovingkindness and tender mercy (Psalm 103:2 - 4 AMP).

Who his self bare our sins in his own body on the tree, that we, being dead to sins, should live unto righteousness: by whose stripes ye were healed (1 Peter 2:24 KJV).

"Death is swallowed up in victory (vanquished forever). 55 O death, where is your victory? O death, where is your sting?" 56 The sting of death is sin, and the power of sin [by which it brings death] is the law; 57 but thanks be to God, who gives us the victory [as conquerors] through our Lord Jesus Christ (1 Corinthians 15:54 - 56 AMP).

It Is Finished

After this, Jesus, knowing that all was now finished, said in fulfillment of the Scripture, "I am thirsty." 29 A jar full of sour wine was placed there; so they put a sponge soaked in the sour wine on [a branch of] hyssop and held it to His mouth. 30 When Jesus had received the sour wine, He said, "It is finished!" And He bowed His head and [voluntarily] gave up His spirit (John 19:28 - 30 AMP).

Tetelesti: It is finished

The Sacrifice is Accomplished (Hebrews 9:12, 26).

He went once for and all into the Holy Place [the Holy of Holies of heaven, into the presence of God], and not through the blood of goats and calves, but through own blood, having obtained and secured eternal redemption [that is, the salvation of all who personally believe in Him as Savior]. 26 Otherwise, He would have needed to suffer over and over since the foundation of the world; but now once for all at the consummation of the ages He has appeared and been publicly manifested to put away sin by the sacrifice of Himself (Hebrews 9:12, 26 AMP).

The Work is Complete (Luke 19:10).

For the Son of Man has come to seek and to save that which was lost (Luke 19:10 AMP).

The Debt is Paid in Full (Hebrews 10:12 - 13; 16).

Whereas Christ, having offered the one sacrifice [the all-sufficient sacrifice of Himself] for sins for all time, sat down [signifying the completion of atonement for sin] at the right hand of God [the position of honor], 13 waiting from that time onward until his enemies are made a footstool for His feet. 16 "This is the covenant that I will make with them after those days, says the Lord: I will imprint My laws upon their heart, and on their mind, I will inscribe them [producing an inward change]" (Hebrews 10:12 - 13; 16 AMP).

EVEN THE DARKEST NIGHT WILL END

What Will I Do
Anoint with Oil
Is anyone among you sick? He must call for the elders (spiritual leaders) of the church and they are to pray over him, anointing him with oil in the name of the Lord; 15 and the prayer of faith will restore the one who is sick, and the Lord will raise him; and if he has committed sins, he will be forgiven. 16 Therefore, confess your sins to one another [your false steps, your offenses], and pray for one another, that you may be healed and restored. The heartfelt and persistent prayer of a righteous man (believer) can accomplish much [when put into action and made effective by God—it is dynamic and can have tremendous power] (James 5:14-16 AMP).

Lord's Supper
For I received from the Lord Himself that [instruction] which I passed on to you, that the Lord Jesus on the night in which He was betrayed took bread; 24 and when He had given thanks, He broke it and said, "This is (represents) My body, which is [offered as a sacrifice] for you. Do this in [affectionate] remembrance of Me." 25 In the same way, after supper He took the cup, saying, "This cup is the new covenant [ratified and established] in My blood; do this, as often as you drink it, in [affectionate] remembrance of Me." 26 For every time you eat this bread and drink this cup, you are [symbolically] proclaiming [the fact of] the Lord's death until He comes [again] (1 Corinthians 11:23 - 26 AMP).

Speak Directly to Satan
Listen carefully: I have given you authority [that you now possess] to tread on serpents and scorpions, and [the ability to exercise authority] over all the power of the enemy (Satan); and nothing will [in any way] harm you (Luke 10:19 AMP).

I speak with boldness, power, and authority with the permission of Jesus Christ. Satan, I do not receive your report. Take it back because it does not belong to the Perry household. We are covered by the precious blood and awesome sacrifice of Jesus Christ, our Lord, and Savior.

SEYMOND PERRY, SR.

Therefore, we are already healed, resisting sickness, injury and disease. Because of the anointing of God in and on our lives, Satan, you must flee now in Jesus' name. Every created thing must respond to and obey the written and spoken Word of God. I have spoken His Word and Cancer; you and all of your workers must obey. You have no place or space in our home or your mind. We have already won the victory for He forever declares that "It Is Finished!" We call you out by name, Satan, you are our sworn enemy and we treat you as such. Get out now in Jesus' name. We thank you Father God for the victory that is already ours in Jesus' name.

EVEN THE DARKEST NIGHT WILL END

Letter to My Job (4/26/2021)

I want to thank each of you for your patience, understanding, and prayers during this difficult and challenging time. I wanted to provide you with some information concerning my son's condition and my plans. After 15 days, my son is no longer in ICU, which is a great improvement in his condition. Although things are better, we are not "out of the woods yet." It has taken great spiritual warfare to get him to this point and I am sure that it will take even more for him to receive his complete and total healing. With that in mind, I will not be returning to work until my son comes home. Although this is a sacrifice, it is one that I willingly and gladly make for the life and well-being of my son. I do not know exactly when he will be discharged (this could be in 2 weeks or 2 months), but I plan to keep his faith strong throughout the entire process. Once again, thank you all so much for everything. I love you with the love of Jesus and together we will make it to the other side.

SEYMOND PERRY, SR.

Lessons Taught While in Hospital
ABC's of Faith (4/22/21)
A - Ask (Mark 11:24)
B - Believe (Mark 11:21 - 24)
C - Confess (Mark 11:23 & 2 Corinthians 4:13)
D - Demonstration (Mark 2:5)
E - Endurance (Mark 5:25 - 34)

- *Example: Woman with the issue of blood*

As Your Soul Prospers (3 John 2)

- *God wants you to succeed and be financially prosperous (Psalm 35:27)*
- *God wants you to be physically healthy*

These areas of your life grow and develop in proportion to the development of your soul.
You are a three-part being: spirit, soul, and body.

- *Your body is your vehicle.*
- *Your spirit is your engine.*
- *Your soul is your navigation system.*

We are going to develop your soul. Your soul is comprised of:

- *Mind: Thought Life (Philippians 4:6 - 9)*

- *Will: Choice (Deuteronomy 24:15)*

- *Intellect: Smart (Proverbs 3:5)*

  ○ *You can learn how to take better care of your body.*

EVEN THE DARKEST NIGHT WILL END

- *Imagination: Extensively dwelling on a thought. This can work for or against us.*

- *Emotions: How you feel (Luke 12:32)*

  ○ *You can take charge of your emotions (2 Corinthians 10:4 - 5).*

The Passover: Exodus 12 (4/24/21)

- *Jesus, Our Passover Lamb (1 Corinthians 5:6 - 7)*
- *(John 1:29)*
- *We Overcome (Revelations 12:11)*

I shall live and not die (Psalm 118:17)
The Importance of the Blood of Jesus (Revelations 12:11)

- *In the natural world and the Bible, blood is a source and symbol of life (Leviticus 17:14).*

- *Blood is mentioned often in the Old Testament, as the Old Testament points to the coming sacrifice (Jesus).*

- *Blood is key to the Passover (Exodus 12).*

- *On The Day of Atonement (Yom Kippur), the high priest would bring blood for the sins of the people.*

- *The wages of sin is death (Romans 6:23).*

- *Forgiveness through blood (Hebrews 9:22)*

Animal and human blood is limited. We need a perfect sacrifice.
Jesus' blood becomes and is the foundation of our relationship with God (Luke 22:20).

SEYMOND PERRY, SR.

The Blood:

- *Redeems us (Ephesians 1:7)*
- *Reconciles us (Romans 3:25)*
- *Ransoms us (1 Peter 1:18 - 19)*
- *Cleans us (1 John 1:7)*
- *Forgives us (Hebrews 9:22)*
- *Frees us (Revelations 1:5)*
- *Justifies us (Romans 5:9)*
- *Cleans our conscience (Hebrews 9:13 - 14)*
- *Sanctifies us (Hebrews 13:12)*
- *Allows access to the Father (Ephesians 2:13)*
- *Gives us peace (Colossians 1:19 - 20)*
- *Overcome the enemy (Revelations 12:11)*

The ABCs of Faith: In Depth (5/3/21)
The Importance of Asking

- *If you want something, it may or may not get done. If you initiate the process by asking, you are more likely to receive your request.*

- *(Ezekiel 22:29 - 31): The Lord does not just do things on the earth. He is looking for a human that will surrender and do His will.*

- *(Genesis 1:26 - 27): God has given us dominion and authority over the earth. What we permit and allow is what will happen.*

- *For God to get involved in our affairs, we must invite Him in. We invite Him by asking.*

- *We must ask to begin the faith process.*

EVEN THE DARKEST NIGHT WILL END

Examples of Asking:

- *(Psalm 34:4 & 6): I sought the Lord - I asked; I cried - I asked.*
- *(Matthew 21:22): Ask*
- *(John 15:7): Ask*
- *(Matthew 7:7 - 8): A.S.K.*

Believe When You Ask - Have Faith When You Ask (5/4/21) *(Mark 11:24)*

- *It is crucial that you must have*

- *Usually, we ask and try to develop faith later.*

- *Why would you ask for something if you did not believe it would happen? You must have faith.*

- *How you can develop this kind of faith (Romans 10:17)?*

- *We are currently believing in healing. {The Word of God must be confessed as often as possible.}*

    o *Isaiah 53:5*

    o *Psalm 103:1-5*

    o *Matthew 8:5-8*

    o *Psalm 41:3*

    o *Psalm 30:2*

Confession: Your Tongue is Your Biggest Weapon: James 3:2 - 12 (5/5/21)

SEYMOND PERRY, SR.

- *Everything is created with Words (Sound): Genesis 1:3*

- *Humanity is created in the image and likeness of God (Genesis 1:27)*

  o *3 part being: spirit, soul, body*

- *If you are created in God's image, you create your world the same way He did, with words.*

- *If we want the life God promised, we will speak His Word.*

- *What you say is a direct reflection of what's in your heart and what you believe (Luke 6:45; Proverbs 4:23; Matthew 12:34).*

- *When you believe you will be found speaking (2 Corinthians 4:13).*

- *We Confess Healing (James 5:14; Mark 9:23; Psalm 41:3; Luke 8:50).*

Faith Can Be Seen/An Act to Demonstrate Your Faith: Matthew 9:2; James 2:26 (5/6/21)

- *Faith can be seen. When someone is operating in true faith, you will see them take action based on that belief.*

- *(James 4:7) - Submit, Resist, the enemy will flee*
- *(Mark 5:25-34) - Women with the issue blood*
- *(Luke 17:11-19) - 10 Lepers healed*
- *(Acts 9:32-35) - Aeneas healed*

What will be your demonstration of faith?
Scriptures on healing?

EVEN THE DARKEST NIGHT WILL END

- *Exodus 15:26*
- *Jeremiah 33:6*
- *Luke 8:50*
- *1 Peter 2:24*
- *Proverbs 4:20-22*

Works Cited

◈ The Holy Bible

◈ **How to Really Love Your Child: Dr. Ross Campbell - Books: 1980**

◈ (The Prayer Ministry of The Church: Watchman Nee - Christian Fellowship Publishers, Inc. - 1973).

◈ Oswald Chambers

◈ The Noticer: Andy Andrew - W. Publishing 2009

◈ The Expeditionary Man: Rich Wagner (Zondervan - 2008)

◈ Look Homeward, Angel - Thomas Wolfe (1929)

◈ From Faith to Faith: Watchman Nee - Christian Fellowship Publishers, Inc.: 1984

◈ **Battling, Brave or Victim: Why the Language of Cancer Matters**
https://breastcancernow.org/about-us/news-personal-stories/battling-brave-or-victim-why-language-cancer-matters

◈ **When Your Child Has Cancer**
https://www.cancer.org/treatment/children-and-cancer/when-your-child-has-cancer.html
-Sachin Ramdas Bharatiya

SEYMOND PERRY, SR.

◈ PTSD Divorce Rate

https://alliancelg.com/ptsd-divorce-rate/#:~:text=The%20symptoms%20of%20post%2Dtraumatic,issues[1]%20and%20help%20their%20partner

---

1. https://alliancelg.com/ptsd-divorce-rate/#_853ae90f0351324bd73ea615e6487517__4c761f170e016836ff84498202b99827__853ae90f0351324bd73ea615e6487517_text_43ec3e5dee6e706af7766fffea512721_The_0bcef9c45bd8a48eda1b26eb0c61c869_20symptoms_0bcef9c45bd8a48eda1b26eb0c61c869_20of_0bcef9c45bd8a48eda1b26eb0c61c869_20post_0bcef9c45bd8a48eda1b26eb0c61c869_2Dtraumatic_c0cb5f0fcf239ab3d9c1fcd31fff1efc_issues

About the Author

Author Seymond Perry, Sr. is a dedicated family man, a teacher, and a minister who has a passion for sharing the wisdom and the word of God. With 20 years of experience in teaching, Seymond has a unique ability to communicate complex ideas in a way that is easy to understand. He is a devoted father and husband, and his experiences as a family man have provided him with valuable insights into the human condition. As a minister, Seymond is committed to spreading the message of God's love and grace to all those who will listen. His writing is an extension of his ministry, as he seeks to share the wisdom he has gained through his life experiences and his faith with others.

Read more at https://themastersrabbi.com/.

CPSIA information can be obtained
at www.ICGtesting.com
Printed in the USA
JSHW031354120323
38820JS00003B/141